101 AMAZING USES for APPLE CiDER ViNEGAR

SOOTHE AN UPSET STOMACH, GET MORE ENERGY, WASH OUT CAT URINE, AND 98 MORE!

Susan Branson

CONTENTS

INTRODUCTION

WHAT IS APPLE CIDER VINEGAR?

Apple cider vinegar is a sour liquid made from apples. The process begins when fresh apples are crushed, releasing the juices. Yeast is added to begin the process of fermentation in which the sugars in the apples are converted to alcohol as they are consumed by the yeast for energy. Bacteria are then added to the alcohol solution to further oxidize the alcohol into acetic acid. Acetic acid is what gives apple cider vinegar its distinctive tart, biting odor and flavor. Fermentation usually takes place over weeks or months. Commercial vinegar is made in wooden barrels to boost the natural fermentation process. Glass jars are more practical for home use, however, and many have successfully made apple cider vinegar on their own. It's best to use organic apples to avoid a heavy load of pesticide residue in the finished product.

Pasteurization is not required because the acidity of the vinegar—usually 5 percent in commercial brands—is enough to prevent any unhealthy microbes from developing. In fact, the raw, unfiltered form is recommended for therapeutic use. Cloudy strands can be seen at the bottom of the bottle which, when shaken, turn the vinegar murky. These strands are known as the Mother and are made up of protein, raw enzymes, and healthy bacteria. Much of the vinegar sold in the grocery stores looks clear and crisp. This has been pasteurized and filtered, and the Mother has been removed. But this vinegar is also very valuable and has many uses in beauty regimens and home products.

SEVEN THOUSAND YEARS OF THANKS FOR APPLE CIDER VINEGAR.

Who gets the credit for making the first vinegar is open for debate. Legend has it that seven thousand years ago, an observant courtier in Babylonia noticed unattended grape juice had turned into wine. What a discovery! This led to the eventual production of vinegar, which the Babylonians flavored with honey, fruit, and malt then sold for consumption and as a preservative. Hippocrates is the first who documented vinegar as a medicine in 400 BC by using it to cleanse wounds. He also mixed it with honey to combat coughs and colds. It is even mentioned in both the Old and New Testaments as a medicine, a drink, and a flavoring agent for food. Sung Tse, the creator of forensic medicine in the tenth century, advised washing hands with sulfur and vinegar to avoid infection during autopsies.[1] Clearly, he felt vinegar had antimicrobial properties. In the eighteenth century, vinegar's popularity had increased and was used by US medical doctors to treat a variety of illnesses including croup, gout, and dysentery.[2]

Today, apple cider vinegar is wildly popular, and its appeal stems from its vast array of applications. It is used therapeutically to improve health by managing symptoms and assisting the body in fighting diseases. The beauty industry uses the prime ingredients in apple cider vinegar to improve the overall look and feel of the skin's tone, the hair's shine, and the mouth's smile. It cleans and disinfects the home, cutting down on chemical-laden products. Apple cider vinegar is good for the body, inside and out, and good for the home, top to bottom.

WHAT IS SO GOOD ABOUT APPLE CIDER VINEGAR?

Acetic acid is the main component of apple cider vinegar, as in all vinegars. It composes roughly 5 percent of the vinegar's content, although this number can vary between 3 and 9 percent. Many of the therapeutic claims stem from the antibacterial and antifungal properties of acetic acid, which protect the body from invasion and infection by a multitude of microbes. The phenolic acids in apple cider vinegar contain these properties, too, and are also known antivirals, antioxidants, antihistamines, and astringents. Some, like gallic acid, have even been shown to be cytotoxic and destroy cancer cells. Malic acid has many uses in enhancing the skin's natural beauty, and it—like the other acids present in apple cider vinegar— protects against pathogens.

The healing properties of apple cider vinegar do not come from its abundant nutrients, as many claims argue. Minerals like potassium, calcium, and the soluble fiber pectin are touted as the source of many of apple cider vinegar's therapeutic benefits. A few nutritional labels report between 11 milligrams and 15 milligrams of potassium in 1 tablespoon (the recommended dietary allowance of potassium is 4700 milligrams per day for adults), but most brands do not report any measurable levels. One study analyzed the mineral content of raw, unfiltered apple cider vinegar and found trace amounts of some minerals but absolutely no potassium.[3] The minerals present were in such small amounts that they were practically negligible in terms of nutritional or therapeutic value. The study also detected small amounts of carbohydrates, which could conceivably be pectin, but again, the amounts range from 0.022 grams to 0.103 grams per tablespoon. Doses in the range of 6 grams (7/10 tablespoon) to 30 grams (3 3/5 tablespoons) of powdered pectin a day are recommended to see the benefits on digestion and blood cholesterol.[4] The standard nutritional analysis of organic, unfiltered, unpasteurized apple cider vinegar with naturally occurring Mother of vinegar shows that it has only 5 calories per tablespoon, making it wonderful as a low-calorie substitute for flavor. However, there are no measureable minerals, vitamins, or protein.[5] This does not support claims that the Mother is rich in enzymes and amino acids, which are proteins. Even in 100 grams of apple cider vinegar, no measurable amounts of minerals, vitamins, or protein were detected.

Another theory about the effectiveness of apple cider vinegar is that it works by changing the pH of the body. When apple cider vinegar is ingested, it creates an alkaline ash in the stomach as it is digested. Some believe that this alkaline ash shifts the pH of the body into a more alkaline state. This is desirable because an acidic state makes the body more open to infection and disease. It is interesting to note that there is also an opposing notion that apple cider vinegar shifts the body into a more acidic state. Foods can change the pH level of the urine; however, the pH level of the blood is strictly controlled by the kidneys and is always maintained at 7.385. Any variations can only happen with certain diseases and can be life threatening if not restored to pH 7.385. Foods cannot change the acidity or alkalinity of the body.

NOT ALL BOTTLES ARE CREATED EQUAL.

In the United States, there are 219 products that contain apple cider vinegar. These come in capsules, tablets, tonics, homeopathic preparations, energy bars, drinks, and powders. There are even shampoos with apple cider vinegar. To obtain the health benefits, most people use either pure apple cider vinegar in liquid form or as tablets and capsules. The FDA does not regulate these supplements, so it's difficult to know exactly what they contain. Eight apple cider vinegar tablet products were tested for their acid content, pH, and microbial growth. Unfortunately, it was determined that considerable variability was found in all parameters tested.[6] This makes it very difficult for the consumer to confidently use these products for health purposes. On the other hand, pure apple cider vinegar is much more likely to contain the active ingredients known to give its healthful benefits because it is standardized for food based on acidity content. Choose a product in a glass bottle that is raw, unfiltered, unpasteurized, and organic. This improves the chances of getting a high-quality, non-GMO product that includes good bacteria left from fermentation without added chemicals or pesticide residue. If you can stand the taste, use pure apple cider vinegar for its benefits. Otherwise, choose a supplement from a reputable company that prioritizes quality control.

HOW MUCH SHOULD I USE?

Natural products often don't come with strict dosages for adults and children. It's important to remember that everything ingested should be done so mindfully and that every food has ingredients that can impact the body in some way. Before taking apple cider vinegar supplements, consult with a healthcare professional and be sure to follow directions on the label. For pure apple cider vinegar, it is recommended that adults take up to 6 tablespoons a day, in divided doses. Many ailments require much less than this, usually between 2 and 3 teaspoons a day. Vinegar is very acidic and can be irritating to mucosal tissues. Always dilute apple cider vinegar with water, and add honey if desired. At this time, there is insufficient evidence to recommend a dosage range for children.

IS TAKING APPLE CIDER VINEGAR SAFE?

Consuming apple cider vinegar in food is safe because the amounts are small and diluted with other ingredients. When taken for medicinal purposes, however, higher amounts are consumed and adverse reactions are more likely. One person developed low potassium levels and osteoporosis after taking a cup of apple cider vinegar a day for six years. In another case, a woman reported pain and tenderness in her larynx after an apple cider vinegar tablet got caught in her throat for thirty minutes.[7] Presumably this was due to the tablet's acid content. Despite these incidences, apple cider vinegar taken in appropriate dosages is likely very safe. That being said, pregnant and breastfeeding women should be cautious because not enough information is known on the effects of apple cider vinegar to the developing fetus or baby.

If medications are taken, apple cider vinegar could possibly interfere with the way they work. Every individual is unique, so unexpected reactions may occur in anyone. Digoxin taken for heart problems can react with large amounts of apple cider vinegar to increase the risk of side effects from the drug. Insulin and excessive apple cider vinegar can decrease potassium levels too much. This can happen with diuretic medication as well. Drugs to lower blood sugar levels combined with too much apple cider vinegar can cause levels to dip too low.

Herbs can have effects on the body, just like medications can. They also have the potential to interact with other foods in a negative way. Apple cider vinegar taken with bitter melon, ginger, fenugreek, or willow bark could cause blood sugar levels to decrease too much. Other herbs combined with apple cider vinegar could deplete potassium levels in the body. Some of these herbs are Canadian hemp roots, licorice, aloe, rhubarb, and senna.[8] Most of these interactions stem from using large amounts of apple cider vinegar. Using appropriate dosages should greatly reduce the chance of any adverse effects.

CHAPTER 1

BOOST YOUR NUTRIENTS AND YOUR MENU

1. FAT SUBSTITUTE

Having a toasted tuna melt oozing with mayonnaise and buttered in margarine is a delicious lunch, but it will have your intake of saturated and trans fats soaring. Saturated fats are known to increase total cholesterol levels in the blood, including the "bad" low-density lipoprotein cholesterol (LDL-C). This can increase the risk of cardiovascular disease and type 2 diabetes. Trans fats not only raise the "bad" cholesterol; they lower the "good," high-density lipoprotein cholesterol (HDL-C). Substituting apple cider vinegar removes the risk introduced by saturated and trans fats and goes further. It decreases "bad" LDL-C and triglyceride levels and increases the "good" HDL-C in the blood.[9] It also has a beneficial effect on blood sugar levels in diabetics.[10]

Next time a tuna melt is on the menu, try mixing apple cider vinegar with olive oil and a sprinkle of dill. Add this to the tuna instead of mayonnaise for a flavorful and healthful sandwich.

2. FOOD PRESERVATIVE

Mold can begin to grow on raspberries very quickly, and green leaf lettuce can decay and wilt before it's consumed. This is not only wasteful but also frustrating when the foods intended for packed lunches or family dinners are no longer useable. To extend the shelf life of fruits and vegetables, try adding 1 cup of apple cider vinegar to 3 cups of water and soaking the produce in the solution for five minutes. Rinse and dry in a spinner or pat dry with a paper towel. Line a container with paper towel, store the produce on top, and put it in the refrigerator.

The vinegar destroys bacteria, viruses, and mold on the surface of the produce so they can't multiply and deteriorate the food. The acidity is thought to break down the microorganism's proteins, thereby destroying them. It works so well that solutions containing 10 percent vinegar are able to reduce bacteria on strawberries by 90 percent and significantly reduce the number of viruses after a two-minute wash.[11] A 4 percent vinegar solution is able to inhibit the growth of *Penicillium chrysogenum*, a common fungus found in indoor environments[12] and whose spores are known human allergens.

3. FOoD TiPS

The versatility of apple cider vinegar in the kitchen will have everyone stocking multiple bottles in their pantries. It can be used in baking and cooking to enhance the process or the final product.

» Adding 1 tablespoon for every 2 1/2 cups of flour will encourage bread to rise, resulting in beautifully fluffy, soft loaves. Just make sure to reduce the amount of water in the recipe by the amount of vinegar used.

» If buttermilk is called for in a recipe and you don't have any on hand, add 1 tablespoon of apple cider vinegar to a cup of milk and let stand for 10 minutes.

» When poaching eggs, adding a little bit of vinegar to the water helps the eggs hold their shape. Even with cracked eggshells, broken while boiling the eggs, egg whites won't seep out if you add apple cider vinegar to the pot.

» Pasta and rice also benefit from a little bit of apple cider vinegar. Instead of salt, the vinegar can be used to prevent noodles from sticking and can make rice fluffier.

» Don't let cheese get dry and moldy. Soak a clean cloth in apple cider vinegar and wrap it around your cheese, then store in a container in the refrigerator. This will preserve the cheese for much longer—hopefully, until it's gone!

4. MEAT TENDERIZER

With all the work that goes into a backyard barbecue feast, ensuring that the star of the show—the meat—is juicy and tender is essential to crown the occasion a success. Some cuts of meat tend to be tough, but with a little help from apple cider vinegar, they can practically melt in the mouth. Marinating meats in apple cider vinegar allows the acid from the vinegar to break down the muscle tissues, soften the fibers by relaxing the protein, and absorb more liquid. The result is a succulent dish. Try this marinade the next time a barbecue is planned.

APPLE CIDER CHICKEN MARINADE
ALLRECIPES.COM

2/3 cup white wine
1/3 cup extra-virgin olive oil
3 tablespoons fresh lemon juice
2 tablespoons apple cider vinegar
3 tablespoons chopped fresh basil
3 tablespoons chopped fresh parsley
1 teaspoon chopped fresh rosemary

1 teaspoon chopped fresh thyme
2 cloves garlic, minced
1 teaspoon freshly ground black pepper
1/2 teaspoon salt

1. Whisk together the white wine, olive oil, lemon juice, vinegar, basil, parsley, rosemary, thyme, garlic, pepper, and salt in a bowl.
2. Marinate chicken in mixture 8 hours or overnight.

5. NO MORE OVERCOOKED BEANS

Despite careful planning, having family members arrive on time for dinner doesn't always happen. Having a last-minute meeting at the office, getting stuck in traffic, or coaching an overtime basketball game are all unplanned events that frequently happen in our lives. But when beans are on the menu and will be ready at six in the evening, what can be done when someone is late and dinner gets put on hold? Slow down the cooking process. This will prevent the beans from overcooking and turning mushy. Adding a few tablespoons of apple cider vinegar to the cooking liquid can do this. The acid in the vinegar slows the softening of the bean's cell walls and makes them more resistant to water absorption. It should be added to the cooking liquid after the beans have already become tender and the desired consistency reached. Make sure not to add the vinegar too early; this may result in tough beans.

NUTRITION

HEALTH

BEAUTY

HOME

6. PICKLING

Long before the days of refrigerators and cold storage, food was preserved in a vinegar or brine solution to extend its lifespan. Pickling in apple cider vinegar creates an acid environment that destroys most bacteria and keeps food edible for several months. As early as 2400 BC, the ancient Mesopotamians are believed to have pickled their food. Ever the forward thinker, Aristotle believed pickled cucumbers had healing effects, and Cleopatra ate pickles to enhance her beauty. Both Julius Caesar and Napoleon fed pickles to their armies to give them strength and good health.[13] Today, pickled produce is abundant in grocery stores, and a quick look at the shelves will reveal jars of cucumbers, asparagus, carrots, peppers, beans, peaches, eggs, and meats, to name a few. The process is not very difficult, and pickling can be done at home. Here is a recipe for pickled grapes.

PICKLED GRAPES
ALLRECIPES.COM

1 pound seedless red grapes
1 1/2 cups apple cider vinegar
1 cup water
1 cup raw sugar
1/2 small red onion, cut into slivers
2 teaspoons yellow mustard seeds
1 teaspoon whole black peppercorns
1 cinnamon stick
1 bay leaf
1 star anise pod
1 whole allspice

1. Remove stems and discard any grapes that aren't firm and unblemished. Place grapes in a quart-size mason jar and set aside.
2. Combine vinegar, water, sugar, onion, mustard seeds, peppercorns, cinnamon stick, bay leaf, star anise pod, and allspice in a saucepan; bring to a boil. Reduce heat to low and simmer until onion is softened—about 10 minutes. Remove saucepan from heat and cool for 15 minutes.
3. Carefully pour cooled liquid over grapes and gently swirl jar to incorporate spices. Cover jar and refrigerate for one day before eating.

NUTRITION

HEALTH

BEAUTY

HOME

CHAPTER 2

BOOST YOUR HEALTH

MANAGING DISEASE

7. ALLERGIES

They can strike in spring when pollen fills the air, at a friend's house when that cute ginger kitten rubs against a leg, or after eating the most satisfying lunch at the local popular seafood restaurant. Allergic reactions can cause minor irritations that result in a stuffy nose, watery eyes, or mild headache, but they can also be so severe as to threaten life. They happen when the immune system reacts to a foreign substance, whether it's swirling through the air, absorbed through the skin, or eaten for lunch. While these substances don't cause a problem for most people, the individual immune system doesn't recognize them in those with allergies. It sees them as unwelcome invaders and launches an attack against them. Specific antibodies are produced for each allergen that identify it as harmful to the body. Every time a person comes in contact with that allergen, the allergic response is activated.

There is no cure for allergies, but there are many over-the-counter and prescription drugs available to help ease symptoms. Among these are antihistamines, decongestants, and corticosteroids. They can cause drowsiness, high blood pressure, insomnia, irritability, restricted urine flow, muscle weakness, fluid retention, and weight gain. And these are just some of the side effects. This seems like trading one set of symptoms for another.

Apple cider vinegar can be ingested to inhibit the release of inflammatory molecules during the allergic response. Gallic acid is a phenolic compound found in apple cider vinegar.[14] It has been found to reduce both systemic and local allergic reactions by blocking the release of histamine and pro-inflammatory cytokines. These molecules promote inflammation and make the symptoms of allergies worse.[15] In the absence of these molecules, the blood vessels no longer dilate, so rashes and itching recede. Mucus production decreases, and productive coughs and runny noses dry up. Bronchial tube constriction eases to relieve coughing and wheezing. And the prevention is easy! Take 2 tablespoons of apple cider vinegar in 1 cup of water up to three times a day to get these benefits.

8. ASTHMA

Asthma is a chronic condition in which the airways leading to the lungs are inflamed. When exposed to triggers (chemicals or situations that impact the body), the airways swell and produce extra mucus. The passageway for air narrows, and breathing becomes more difficult. Symptoms include coughing, shortness of breath, wheezing, and chest pain. Anyone can develop asthma, although some are genetically predisposed to it. Triggers can be allergens, both environmental and food, or other substances like smoke, pollution, or changes in the weather. Learning what your specific triggers are goes a long way in asthma management. Doctors often prescribe controller medications like corticosteroids, long-acting beta agonists, and sometimes leukotriene modifiers to help manage the condition. Short-acting beta agonists are prescribed to quickly relieve symptoms by relaxing and opening the airways.

Gallic acid is a phenolic compound in apple cider vinegar[16] that has been shown to inhibit histamine and pro-inflammatory cytokines that cause inflammation of the airways and mucus production.[17] These compounds trigger reactions that make breathing very difficult, and the asthmatic suffers from wheezing, coughing, and bronchial spasms. By obstructing these compounds, tissue in the airways shrink, mucus is removed, and the flow of air into the lungs in greatly increased. Symptoms subside. Drinking 2 tablespoons of apple cider vinegar in 1 cup of water each day should reduce the inflammatory response of the lungs and bring relief to many. If the taste of the drink is not desirable, sweeten it with honey.

9. ATHEROSCLEROSIS

This is a disease in which plaque builds up inside the arteries, the blood vessels that carry oxygen-rich blood to the body. Plaque collects along the arterial walls and is made up of fat, cholesterol, calcium, and other substances. Over time, the plaque hardens and makes the arterial path smaller. If not treated, blood flow can become so constricted that a heart attack, stroke, or even death may result.

Atherosclerosis is a very common disease and often exists without any outward symptoms. The risk factors include an unhealthy diet, lack of exercise, and smoking. It is not surprising, then, that the main treatment is a change in lifestyle to incorporate healthy choices.

Apple cider vinegar is effective in reducing high blood fat levels. A study in male rats found that a diet containing a 6 percent solution by weight was able to significantly reduce LDL-C (the "bad" cholesterol) and significantly increase HDL-C (the "good" cholesterol). Triglycerides were also lowered.[18] Having elevated levels of "good" cholesterol is important as they pick up the "bad" cholesterol and bring it to the liver. This reduces the levels of LDL-C in the blood and lowers the risk of the "bad" cholesterol being oxidized. Oxidized "bad" cholesterol activates the inflammatory response in the arterial walls and leads to the development of plaque.

The phenolic compounds in apple cider vinegar, particularly the abundant chlorogenic acid, can assist in preventing the "bad" cholesterol from being oxidized.[19] These phenolic compounds are antioxidants and are able to neutralize the free radicals, thereby preventing damage. Apple cider vinegar can improve serum lipid profiles and eliminate the threat of free radicals to reduce the risk of atherosclerosis.

10. BRONCHITIS

Bronchitis is a respiratory disease characterized by the inflammation of the lining of the bronchial airways of the lungs. Acute bronchitis can result from a cold or other respiratory infection, causing the mucous membranes to swell and air pathways to narrow. Chronic bronchitis is more severe and is a constant inflammation of the lining of the bronchial tubes, most often caused by smoking. People with bronchitis have coughing spells and often

NUTRITION

HEALTH

BEAUTY

HOME

NUTRITION

HEALTH

BEAUTY

HOME

cough up mucus. Chest pain, fever, chills, and fatigue are other symptoms. Acute bronchitis often goes away on its own after a short time, while chronic bronchitis persists and often requires cough medicine, asthma inhalers, or antibiotics if a bacterial infection is suspected.

Hippocrates recommended vinegar with honey to treat the symptoms of coughs and cold.[20] Apple cider vinegar contains gallic acid, an acid capable of interfering with the body's natural inflammatory response. Specifically, it works by inhibiting the release of histamine and pro-inflammatory cytokines that cause inflammation of the airways and mucus production.[21] These compounds trigger reactions that make breathing very difficult. By obstructing these compounds, tissues in the airways shrink and mucus is removed. Air can flow freely into and out of the lungs. Vinegar was even used thousands of years ago for respiratory issues.

Bronchitis caused by an infection will also benefit from apple cider vinegar. Acetic acid and the phenolic acids in the vinegar are all antimicrobial compounds and can destroy the source of infection, whether it is bacterial or viral. Try warming a cup of water and adding a tablespoon each of apple cider vinegar and honey to break up congestion and open up the respiratory pathways.

11. CANCEROUS TUMORS

Cells of the body grow, divide, and die. New cells replace the old, and a balance is maintained. Cancer cells grow and divide rapidly and continue to live when the normal cell life cycle is over. They begin to crowd out healthy cells, and the balance is disturbed. Tumors can form. The exact cause of cancer is not understood, but it is thought that both genetic and environmental factors are at play, including toxins, excessive sunlight, radiation, and viruses. Symptoms are dependent on the type and location of the tumor. Common treatments include chemotherapy, radiation, surgery, and medications.

It is difficult to avoid toxins in the environment, so it is wise to take steps to ensure the body has the necessary compounds it needs to prevent tumors from forming. One class of these protective compounds is antioxidants. The phenolic acids in apple cider vinegar are known antioxidants. Consuming phenolic compounds increases antioxidant protection within the body and can reduce cancer risk and the formation of tumors.[22] It is thought that the acetic acid in apple cider vinegar may also possess antitumor effects. Acetic acid breaks down into acetate in the stomach and has been found to significantly reduce rapid cell division of cancerous human colon cells.[23] Tumor development is delayed, enabling more time for detection and treatment. Another study fed vinegar in the diet to tumor-bearing mice for seventy-two days. Tumors were significantly smaller, and the lifespan of these mice was prolonged over mice not fed vinegar.[24] A little apple cider vinegar a day could reduce the risk of developing tumors or slow their progression.

12. CANDIDIASIS

Candidiasis is a fungal infection caused by the yeast-like *Candida* fungus. There are over twenty species of *Candida* that can infect humans, but *Candida albicans* is the most common. These yeasts normally live on the skin and mucous membranes in people and are generally harmless. If conditions in the body shift to create an

NUTRITION

HEALTH

BEAUTY

HOME

environment favorable to *Candida* overgrowth, infections of the mouth, vagina, urinary tract, skin, or stomach can set it. Most causes of *Candida* overgrowth result from certain drugs, pregnancy, bacterial infections, excess weight, or an overburdened immune system. Vaginal yeast infections, white lesions on the tongue or inner cheek, painful cracks in the skin at the corners of the mouth, or crusted skin rashes around the fingers, toes, and groin are symptoms of candidiasis. Antifungal drugs are commonly prescribed for up to two weeks.

Reducing sugar and yeast products in the diet and taking probiotics are popular alternative therapies to getting rid of candidiasis. Apple cider vinegar can be used alongside these practices. A laboratory study applied a 4 percent solution of apple cider vinegar to *Candida* species in varying conditions and times. It demonstrated significant fungicidal properties after thirty minutes of exposure.[25] When apple cider vinegar is ingested, it is rapidly absorbed from the gastrointestinal tract and broken down. In order for the active ingredients to have a fungicidal effect in the body, they need to reach the fungus intact. *Candida* overgrowth often happens in the intestines before spreading out into the body. Halting growth there should stop the spread of the infection. Consuming an enteric-coated apple cider vinegar capsule should allow the active ingredients to work directly on the *Candida* in the intestines. Follow the directions on the capsule's label. If the presence of *Candida albicans* is causing inflammation and redness beneath dentures, soaking them in a 10 percent vinegar solution overnight significantly reduces the amount of yeast and can also reduce swelling and redness.[26] Candidiasis is very common, so consider taking apple cider vinegar as either a preventative measure or as a safe alternative to antifungal drugs.

13. DIABETES

Diabetes is a disease that affects the way the body handles glucose, resulting in high levels of this sugar in the blood. There is type 1 diabetes, in which the pancreas produces little or no insulin, type 2 diabetes, in which the pancreas does produce insulin but the body doesn't use it as well as it should, and gestational diabetes, a form of high blood sugar affecting pregnant women. Some people are genetically predisposed to diabetes, but being overweight is also a risk factor. Feelings of thirst, frequent urination, fatigue, tingling, numbness in the hands or feet, and blurry vision are all signs of diabetes. Managing diabetes involves exercising, improving diet, and monitoring blood glucose levels. For many, daily insulin injections are needed.

The high incidence of diabetes makes finding an easy and natural alternative to manage this disease very desirable. Studies toward this end have uncovered apple cider vinegar as an effective agent in this regard. Four randomized crossover trials in adults with either no diabetes or type 2 diabetes were given 2 teaspoons of vinegar with a bagel and juice. After two hours, the amount of glucose in the blood was effectively reduced by 20 percent compared to placebo.[27] These researchers have also demonstrated an improvement in insulin sensitivity by 19 percent in type 2 diabetic patients and 34 percent in insulin-resistant subjects.[28]

Vinegar may work by delaying the rate of gastric emptying.[29] This would slow the uptake of sugar into the blood and allow the body more time to effectively manage glucose levels. Another theory is that vinegar may prevent the complete digestion of complex

NUTRITION

HEALTH

BEAUTY

HOME

carbohydrates or slow their conversion into sugar. This would mean fewer sugars are present in the blood at any one time, lessening the potential for an influx of too much glucose for the body to handle. Apple cider vinegar, then, may be valuable in controlling blood sugar levels and managing the effects of diabetes in humans.

14. E. COLI POISONING

Escherichia coli is bacteria that normally live in the intestines of humans and animals. Many types of *E. coli* are harmless and are important to the health of the digestive tract. Several species, however, are pathogenic and cause bloody diarrhea, urinary tract infections, anemia, or kidney failure. Contraction of *E. coli* can be made from contact with infected persons or animals or from consuming food or water containing the bacteria. *E. coli* can contaminate meat during processing, and if it is not cooked to 160 degrees Fahrenheit, it can survive and infect the consumer. Sometimes, cows spread the bacteria to their milk as it passes through their udders. If the milk is not pasteurized, the bacteria will continue to live and pose a threat. Even raw fruits and vegetables can have *E. coli* bacteria from contact with contaminated water or persons. Three or four days after ingesting *E. coli*, food poisoning becomes evident as symptoms develop. They usually subside on their own after about a week.

Anyone who has been through an episode of food poisoning understands how absolutely miserable it is. Once an infection is underway, frequent vomiting may make drinking apple cider vinegar impossible. That means prevention is key. Cooking meats to their proper temperature and washing produce to remove any offending pathogens is essential. Apple cider vinegar is an effective, natural, and safe product that can eliminate *E. coli* on food. *E. coli* O157:H7 is one of the common strains infecting humans worldwide. A 0.1 percent concentration of acetic acid, the main component of apple cider vinegar, was found to inhibit the growth of this strain.[30] Other compounds in apple cider vinegar—caffeic acid and p-coumaric acid—have also been shown to inhibit its growth.[31] The acid in vinegar crosses the bacterial cell membrane and causes a release of protons, resulting in cell death.[32] Be sure to wash all produce with a diluted solution of apple cider vinegar to decrease the potential for *E. coli* food poisoning. The solution should be three parts water to one part vinegar. Let the produce sit in this solution for about ten minutes, then rinse with clean water.

15. ESOPHAGEAL CANCER

The long, hollow tube that runs from the throat to the stomach is the esophagus. It carries food from the mouth to the stomach for digestion. When the cells that line this tube mutate and begin to divide in an uncontrolled way, cancer of the esophagus can develop. These cells can accumulate into tumors that continue to grow and can invade nearby tissues or spread to other parts of the body. During the early stages, no symptoms are noticed. As it progresses, difficulty swallowing, unintentional weight loss, chest pain, indigestion, or hoarseness may occur. Smoking and poorly controlled long-term acid reflux are significant risk factors. Surgery is commonly performed to remove the tumor with or without chemotherapy and radiation. Side effects of these treatments include infection, bleeding, painful swallowing, or accidental damage to nearby organs.

If the disease is already present, following the advice of a primary care physician or specialist is recommended. For those who are at high risk, daily consumption of apple cider vinegar can help reduce that risk. A case-controlled study in China showed that vinegar had a protective effect and decreased the chance of developing esophageal cancer.[33] As a preventive measure, take 1 tablespoon of apple cider vinegar diluted in water each day.

16. FATTY LIVER (STEATOSIS)

This disease is very common and is characterized by an accumulation of fat in the liver cells. It is caused when liver cells are damaged from alcohol (alcoholic steatosis), metabolic dysfunction, or insulin resistance (nonalcoholic steatosis). Those at risk have high blood pressure, high blood lipids, type 2 diabetes, abnormal glucose tolerance, or are overweight or drink alcohol to excess. If the disease is caused by alcohol, abstinence can reverse it. Otherwise, the combination of a healthy diet and exercise is recommended to better control weight, diabetes, and cardiovascular health.

Type 2 diabetes and impaired glucose tolerance can cause periods of too much glucose in the blood. The liver takes up glucose and stores it as glycogen, but when there is too much glucose in the blood, it converts it into fat. When the body's fat stores are full, the liver will hang on to the excess fat itself. By taking apple cider vinegar daily with meals, blood glucose levels can be reduced by 20 percent[34] and insulin sensitivity improved by 19 percent.[35] By decreasing blood sugar levels, the liver has less chance of storing glucose as fat in its own cells.

Ingesting apple cider vinegar can also reduce blood fat levels. A study in rats showed 10 milliliters of vinegar taken with a high-cholesterol diet significantly reduced LDL-C, total cholesterols, and oxidized LDL-C in the blood.[36] This reduction in serum lipids can lighten the fat load stored in the liver. An interesting benefit of consuming apple cider vinegar is that it decreases appetite and can reduce the calories ingested by people trying to lose weight. The result could be an improved steatosis outlook.

In one study, twelve healthy volunteers were each fed white bread for breakfast. One meal was bread alone, and the other meals included bread with various levels of acetic acid in vinegar. Study participants reported feeling full after consuming bread with vinegar as compared to the meal with no vinegar. This feeling of fullness was directly related to the level of acetic acid in the vinegar.[37] Apple cider vinegar taken with meals can satisfy the appetite and has been reported to decrease calorie intake by approximately 200 to 275 calories.[38] It can be used to help manage the risks that lead to nonalcoholic steatosis. To take advantage of these results, try taking 1 tablespoon in a cup of water before each meal.

17. FIBROMYALGIA

This disorder is characterized by widespread muscle pain and tenderness. It is thought that the brains of those with fibromyalgia process pain signals differently and amplify painful sensations. Sleep is often disrupted, fatigue constant, memory impaired, and mood altered. Symptoms can occur gradually over time or be triggered by severe stress, infection, surgery, or trauma. Those suffering from fibromyalgia can take medications for pain or antidepressants to help with sleep. As with any medications, side effects are not uncommon. Nausea, rashes, upset stomach, weight gain, and sexual problems are just a few.

Malic acid is a constituent of apple cider vinegar. It is commonly known to increase energy and reduce pain; pain and fatigue are the two most prevalent symptoms of fibromyalgia. Apple cider vinegar, taken daily, may benefit systemic pain and fatigue within a few days. Fifteen fibromyalgia patients were treated with a combination of malic acid and magnesium over eight weeks. Mood was elevated[39] and pain and tenderness were significantly improved over patients receiving placebo.[40] The malic acid and magnesium work together to metabolize carbohydrates to provide energy for the body and reduce fatigue and pain.

Apple cider vinegar also increases iron absorption. Iron is needed in the body to deliver oxygen to cells and is used to boost energy, mood, and concentration. Making a spinach salad with an apple cider vinaigrette would be a great way to get both magnesium and malic acid to assist in managing the symptoms of fibromyalgia.

APPLE CIDER VINAIGRETTE

1/2 cup apple cider vinegar
1/4 cup olive oil
2 teaspoons honey mustard
1 teaspoon crushed garlic
1/4 teaspoon salt

1. Mix all ingredients together.
2. Shake or stir vinaigrette before pouring over salad to recombine any ingredients that have separated.

18. GINGIVITIS

Gingiva is the part of the gum around the base of the teeth that becomes diseased and falls prey to gingivitis. The gums tend to bleed easily, become puffy, and turn from pink to red. They begin to recede, and tooth decay sets in. Gingivitis is caused when hardened plaque, called tartar, forms below and above the gum line. Tartar is full of bacteria, and it is the bacteria that begin the infection. Plaque is formed daily on the teeth, but it can easily be removed through daily brushing and flossing. If it is left to harden into tartar, it is much harder to eliminate. This disease is common, and symptoms are often mild, so most people don't know they have it. Professional teeth cleaning is needed, followed by a good oral hygiene routine at home.

An effective preventative for gingivitis is to use apple cider vinegar in a mouthwash just before brushing. Add 1 tablespoon to 1/2 cup water and swirl around the mouth for thirty seconds. Follow by brushing with toothpaste or baking soda. Apple cider vinegar is very acidic and can erode the tooth's enamel. For this reason, never use it undiluted. It works by destroying the bacteria in the mouth, causing gingivitis. Acetic acid and the phenolic acids in vinegar are able to cross the bacterial cell membranes and cause major destruction and death. One of the phenolic compounds, gallic acid, is a known anti-inflammatory and can reduce the redness and swelling caused by the infection. This will heal the mouth and clear up the infection more quickly. Apple cider vinegar's use would be a safe and inexpensive addition to an oral hygiene routine for the prevention and treatment of gingivitis.

NUTRITION

HEALTH

BEAUTY

HOME

19. GOUT

Gout is a form of arthritis that causes severe pain, tenderness, and swelling in joints, most commonly at the base of the big toe. An attack of gout can come on suddenly and happen over and over unless treated. It is caused when too much uric acid in the blood builds up to the point that uric acid crystals are formed in the joints. These crystals are sharp and needlelike, causing pain, redness, and swelling. Medications are used to treat acute attacks and prevent future attacks. They include nonsteroidal anti-inflammatories, corticosteroids, and colchicine to reduce pain and inflammation. Other medications to block uric acid production or increase its removal can also be prescribed for patients in severe pain. Side effects include stomach pain, nausea, vomiting, diarrhea, mood changes, rashes, and kidney stones.

Apple cider vinegar contains gallic acid, which is touted as having properties that relieve pain and inflammation, the two common symptoms of gout.[41] Its action is through inhibiting enzymes involved in the inflammatory response. Tissue swelling and tenderness decrease, alleviating pressure on the nerves and reducing pain.

In his book *Alkalize or Die*, Dr. Theodore Baroody declares that an acidic pH balance in the body can cause gout, but by shifting the body back into an alkaline state, gout should disappear and not come back. He goes on to say that drinking apple cider vinegar can help create this shift. Then, the body can break up uric acid crystals in the joints and prevent them from reforming. He cautions that inflammation may initially increase as the uric acid crystals dissolve but that all symptoms should dissipate within a few weeks.[42]

While there is little doubt for many people that apple cider vinegar is very effective in treating gout, the exact mechanism by which it does so has not been thoroughly investigated. It should be mentioned that there is no scientific evidence supporting the theory that foods can alter the pH level of the body. Acidic foods can increase the acidity of the urine, but the body tightly regulates blood pH to 7.385 regardless of the foods eaten.

20. GRANuLAR MYRINGITIS

This disease is a chronic infection in the outer layers of skin of the eardrum. It is characterized by the formation of granulation tissue—new connective tissue that grows on the surface of a wound. It can have a bumpy appearance and be bright pink or red in color; this is healthy tissue. However, the wounded tissue underneath is inflamed and swollen with fluid. Bacteria or fungus invade the ear and infect the tissue of the eardrum. Poor hygiene, swimming, high ambient temperatures, or local irritations may aggravate the condition. With this condition, there is little or no pain and sometimes no symptoms are reported. More often, however, patients complain of a foul-smelling discharge from the infected ear, mild hearing impairment, or a feeling of inner ear fullness. To treat the infection, antibiotics, antifungals, and steroids are prescribed. While taking these medications is effective in treating granular myringitis, the patient may develop hives, rashes, stinging, or further skin irritation.

As an alternative treatment to these medications, a diluted solution of apple cider vinegar can be used to manage granular myringitis. One study compared topical antibiotic drops to a diluted vinegar wash in the treatment of thirty patients with chronic granular myringitis. A dry ear was achieved in six weeks in those receiving the diluted vinegar, while it took six months in patients using topical antibiotics.[43] Acetic acid and the phenolic acids in the vinegar have the ability to kill these pathogens by crossing their cell membranes and disrupting metabolic functions. Caution must be taken to adequately dilute the vinegar with an equal amount of 85 percent rubbing alcohol to ensure the acids do not irritate the inflamed tissue.

21. HIGH CHOLESTEROL

Cholesterol is a waxy, fat-like substance found in cells. It is necessary for the body to make vitamin D, hormones, and bile acids that help digest food. We produce cholesterol on our own, but we also get it in saturated fat and cholesterol-laden foods. It comes in two forms: the good and the bad. High cholesterol is when there are high levels of cholesterol in the blood, both good and bad. When there is too much of the bad cholesterol in the body, however, it can build up in the arteries and increase the chances of getting coronary heart disease. Plaque containing cholesterol builds up inside the arteries and causes partial or full blockage, leading to narrowing and hardening of the arteries. This can lead to a heart attack or stroke. Statins are drugs commonly prescribed to lower the bad blood cholesterol. Taking statins can cause intestinal problems and muscle inflammation.

Cholesterol levels respond well to changes in diet. Eating foods low in saturated fats and reducing intake of animal products—which are the contributors of cholesterol in the diet—will do wonders. Apple cider vinegar has been studied for its effect on blood fat levels and was found to be effective. A study in male rats found that a diet containing a 6 percent apple cider vinegar solution by weight was able to significantly reduce LDL-C (the "bad" cholesterol) and significantly increase HDL-C (the "good" cholesterol). Triglycerides were also lowered.[44, 45] Consuming apple cider vinegar appears to be effective in managing cholesterol and reducing the risk of coronary heart disease.

22. HYPERGLYCEMIA

This is high blood sugar. Hyperglycemia happens when the body doesn't produce insulin, produces too little insulin, or can't properly use the insulin it secretes so that cells are unable to take up the sugar from the blood. It is often associated with diabetes, but non-diabetics can develop hyperglycemia from a surge of hormones, stress, or illness. Lowering blood sugar is essential to prevent complications affecting the eyes, kidneys, heart, and nerves. Severe hyperglycemia can lead to a life-threatening diabetic coma. This condition develops slowly, and early signs include increased thirst, frequent urination, fatigue, and headache. As it progresses, weakness, confusion, nausea, vomiting, and fruity-smelling breath are common. Hyperglycemia can be managed with a combination of drugs, exercise, and proper diet.

Two tablespoons of apple cider vinegar, taken before bed, were shown to lower blood sugar levels in diabetics by 4 or 6 percent overnight.[46] This reduction in fasting glucose by vinegar is significant for those experiencing the dawn syndrome—an abnormal rise in blood glucose levels early in the morning. Four randomized crossover trials in adults with either no diabetes or type 2 diabetes were given 2 teaspoons of vinegar with a bagel and juice. After two hours, the amount of glucose in the blood was effectively reduced by 20 percent compared to placebo.[47] While acetic acid is thought to be responsible for much of apple cider vinegar's effect on glucose, another of its constituents may be involved, too. Chlorogenic acid, one of apple cider vinegar's phenolic acids, has been found to significantly reduce glucose concentrations in overweight men.[48] Vinegar may work by delaying the rate of gastric emptying.[49] This would slow the uptake of sugar into the blood and allow the body more time to effectively manage glucose levels. Another theory is that vinegar may prevent the complete digestion of complex carbohydrates or slow their conversion into sugar. This would mean fewer sugars are present in the blood at any one time, lessening the potential for an influx of too much glucose for the body to handle. A daily dose of apple cider vinegar could lower glucose levels in both diabetics and nondiabetics.

23. HYPERTENSION

The force exerted against arterial walls as blood flows through them determines blood pressure. The pressure is measured in the arteries when the heart contracts (systolic) and when the heart is at rest (diastolic). It is determined by how much blood the heart pumps and the resistance it encounters as it flows through the arteries. Blood pressure sustained above 140/90 mmhg (millimeters of mercury) is considered high, and hypertension results. This condition develops slowly over time, and many people have it without knowing. It can damage blood vessels and the heart. If left untreated, it can lead to heart attack and stroke. Primary hypertension doesn't have any identifiable cause, although obesity, smoking, poor diet, lack of exercise, and high salt intake are some commonly seen risk factors. Secondary hypertension has an underlying cause and could result from drugs or certain medications, alcohol abuse, thyroid problems, or kidney issues. Hypertension responds well to changes in lifestyle. Exercising more, eating a nutrient-rich diet, reducing stress, and quitting smoking and alcohol consumption should bring blood pressure down. There are many drugs available to lower blood pressure, including thiazide diuretics to reduce blood volume, beta blockers to slow down the heart rate, ACE inhibitors to block the action of some hormones that regulate blood pressure, calcium channel blockers, and renin inhibitors to widen the arteries. All these medications come with significant side effects like diarrhea, fatigue, dizziness, nausea, erectile dysfunction, and headaches.

Changes in lifestyle should be the first line of defense against high blood pressure. If additional measures are needed, try including 2 teaspoons of apple cider vinegar in the diet each day before relying on any of the medications described above. Blood pressure could be lowered without having to endure any of the many side effects of these drugs. A double-blind placebo-controlled study tested two vinegar and dried bonito- (tuna-) containing water preparations in normal to moderately hypertensive patients. They found that both solutions significantly decreased systolic and diastolic blood pressure.[50] Another study found that acetic acid (the main component of apple cider vinegar) significantly reduced blood pressure by decreasing compounds that constrict the arteries and increase blood volume, both of which lead to higher blood pressure.[51] Apple cider vinegar also contains chlorogenic acid, which was proven to reduce blood pressure in mildly hypertensive humans without any side effects.[52]

24. KIDNEY INFECTION

A kidney infection is actually a specific type of urinary tract infection. Bacteria enter the body from the skin around the urethra, the tube that carries urine out of the body from the bladder. The bacteria migrate up the urethra, the bladder, and ureters (the tubes that carry urine from the kidneys to the bladder) to reach the kidneys. Here the bacteria begin to multiply, and the infection takes hold. The bacteria can also spread through the blood to the kidneys from an infection elsewhere in the body. This route of infection, however, is much less common. A kidney infection needs prompt medical attention because it can spread to the blood and cause life-threatening complications. It may be accompanied by fever, backache, abdominal pain, frequent urination, or urine that smells bad, is cloudy, or has blood or pus in it. Antibiotics are the first line of defense for kidney infections.

The acetic acid and phenolic acids in apple cider vinegar have the ability to destroy bacteria. One of the common bacteria-causing kidney infections is *E. coli*. These bacteria can transfer from the stool to the skin to the urethra. Apple cider vinegar is an effective, natural, and safe product that can eliminate *E. coli*. A 0.1 percent concentration of acetic acid was found to inhibit the growth *E. coli*.[53] The phenolic acids—caffeic acid and *p*-Coumaric acid—have also been found to inhibit its growth as well as the growth of *Klebsiella pneumoniae*,[54] another bacteria commonly responsible for kidney infections. The acid in vinegar crosses the bacterial cell membranes and causes a release of protons, resulting in cell death. If a person is prone to urinary tract infections, washing the area between the anus and urethra with a cotton ball soaked in apple cider vinegar should destroy any bacteria that have adhered to the skin. This should be done after a bowel movement and careful cleaning. Another way to avoid urinary tract infections, which lead to kidney infections, is to drink 2 tablespoons of apple cider vinegar in 1 cup of water three times a day. This will create a slightly acidic urine environment for the infectious bacteria and discourage its growth.[55] It should be discontinued, however, if voiding is painful or if the infection is severe. The more acidic urine may further irritate the already inflamed and sensitive lining of the bladder and ureters. It is thought that the slight, temporary acidity of the urine created by ingesting apple cider vinegar can work toward preventing a urinary tract infection or stopping one in its early stages. If the condition is advanced, however, a trip to the doctor for a course of antibiotics is recommended.

25. OSTEoPOROSIS

Osteoporosis is a bone disease in which the body can't produce enough new bone to replace old bone removal. The process of bone absorption and replacement happens continuously in the body, but in those with osteoporosis, bone mass decreases over time. A decrease in mass and density results in weakened bones that are more likely to break. It is more common in women than men because women have lower bone masses. Osteoporosis is known as a silent disease because it doesn't produce symptoms and diagnosis is often made after a bone has been broken. This disease runs in families, so if a parent or grandparent had osteoporosis, there is an increased chance the next generation will have it too. Certain diseases and medications can also increase the likelihood of developing osteoporosis. A healthy diet sufficient in bone-producing minerals, weight-bearing exercises, and medication are recommended for management and treatment. Calcium is a mineral in food that is stored in the bones and teeth and is essential to keep them healthy and strong. Bones are constantly being broken down and built up, so calcium moves in and out of the bones during these processes. As the body ages, bones are broken down at a faster rate than they are formed. It is essential that enough calcium is available in the body to incorporate into the manufacture of new bones to prevent osteoporosis.

Apple cider vinegar enhances the absorption of calcium from food, making this essential mineral more available to take part in bone formation. Acetic acid in vinegar is broken down into acetate in the body. Acetate was found to increase calcium absorption in human distal colons and rectums in healthy human subjects.[56] In a rat model, acetic acid not only enhanced calcium absorption but increased its retention as well.[57] Including apple cider vinegar with meals or drinking a solution of 1 tablespoon of apple cider vinegar in 1 cup of water before meals should help increase calcium bioavailability for bone building and decrease the risk of osteoporosis.

26. RHEUMATOID ARTHRITIS

Rheumatoid arthritis is an autoimmune disorder in which the immune system mistakenly attacks its own body tissues. The lining of the joints become painfully swollen, which can lead to bone erosion and joint deformity over time. Symptoms can spread to other non-joint tissues of the body. It's not known what causes this disease, but genetics combined with environmental triggers are suspected. This chronic disease is without a cure and is managed mostly through medications. Nonsteroidal anti-inflammatory drugs, steroids, or disease-modifying antirheumatic drugs can be prescribed to reduce pain, swelling, and joint damage. Possible side effects include digestive problems, liver and kidney damage, heart problems, thinning of bones, diabetes, weight gain, and severe lung infections.

Fortunately, apple cider vinegar can help reduce inflammation and pain associated with rheumatoid arthritis without any of the side effects. Gallic acid, a phenolic compound in apple cider vinegar, has been found to induce death in specialized cells in the joints that cause inflammation in rheumatoid arthritis.[58] This prevents inflammation and swelling in the affected joints, which subsequently alleviates pressure on the nerves and reduces pain. The acetic acid in vinegar enhances calcium absorption to help the body build bone to minimize loss due to bone erosion. Making an apple cider vinegar poultice to wrap around affected joints can be done at home. Heat 1 cup of water with 1/4 cup apple cider vinegar to a comfortable temperature. Soak a clean cloth in the solution, wring out excess liquid, and wrap it over the tender area. Cover with a dry, clean cloth or a plastic bag for fifteen minutes.

NUTRITION

HEALTH

BEAUTY

HOME

27. SALMONELLOSIS

This is a type of food poisoning caused by the *Salmonella* bacteria. It enters the system through contaminated food. This contamination can happen to poultry, beef, milk, eggs, and even vegetables during food processing and handling. *Salmonella* is also found in some pets, such as ducklings, reptiles, hamsters, and other small rodents. Hand washing is recommended after handling these animals to prevent infection. If *Salmonella* poisoning does happen, it usually occurs within twelve to seventy-two hours after it enters the body. Diarrhea, stomach cramps, and fever develop and can last up to a week. They eventually subside without medication.

There is no way to know if produce contains the *Salmonella* bacteria because the food looks and smells normal. The best way to avoid infection is by prevention. Wash all produce in a solution that is one part apple cider vinegar to three parts water. The acid in vinegar crosses the bacterial cell membranes, causing a release of protons and cell death. One of the most common pathogenic *Salmonella* species is *Salmonella typhimurium*. This bacteria was reduced to undetectable levels on vegetables fifteen minutes after an application of vinegar and lemon juice.[59] Cutting boards and countertops can also be breeding grounds for *Salmonella*, especially if used to prepare meats. Spray apple cider vinegar directly onto the surface and let sit for a few minutes. Scrub and rinse with clean water. Be sure to spray the sink, too, in case any live bacteria remains there.

It is conceivable that since the acid in apple cider vinegar kills the bacteria outside the body, it may do so inside the body as well.

When apple cider vinegar is ingested, it is rapidly absorbed from the gastrointestinal tract and broken down. In order for the active ingredients to have a bactericidal effect in the body, they need to reach the bacteria intact. *Salmonella* infection happens in the intestines, so consuming an enteric-coated apple cider vinegar capsule should allow the active ingredients to work directly on the *Salmonella* in the intestines and destroy them. Follow the directions on the label.

28. SHINGLES

Shingles is a viral infection of a nerve area that causes pain and a rash along the skin where the affected nerve lies. It is the same virus responsible for chickenpox. This virus lays dormant at the base of the nerves next to the spinal cord. It can be reactivated years later and travel along the nerves to the skin. It is not known what causes the virus to become active after years of being dormant, but a depressed immune system is thought to be one reason. Usually, only one nerve is affected on one side of the body, but sometimes two or three that are close together can be involved. The chest, abdomen, and upper face are common sites. The band of pain and rash is tender, inflamed, and itchy. Symptoms usually go away in two to four weeks. Painkillers, antidepressants, and anticonvulsants are commonly given to help with nerve pain. Other medications include steroids to help reduce inflammation and antivirals to stop the spread of the virus.

The acetic acid and phenolic acids (*p*-coumaric, gallic, caffeic, and chlorogenic) in apple cider vinegar are all antiviral

NUTRITION

HEALTH

BEAUTY

HOME

compounds. With a cotton ball, apply one part apple cider vinegar to three parts water to the affected area. Let air dry and repeat as needed. Not only does this work in weakening the virus and stopping the spread of the infection, but it also relieves itching. Gallic acid has been shown to inhibit histamine and pro-inflammatory cytokines that cause inflammation.[60] This reduces swelling and allows the skin tissues to relieve pressure on the nerve to reduce pain. A warm bath with 1 cup of apple cider vinegar added should provide relief.

29. SINUSITIS

The hollow air spaces within the bones around the nose are the sinuses. When they become swollen and inflamed, sinusitis develops. The tissues produce thick yellow or green mucus, which drains into the nose or down the back of the throat. Breathing through the nose becomes difficult, and there may be pain, pressure, or tenderness around the eyes or nose that worsens when bending over. Sometimes, the pain extends to the ears, jaws, and teeth. Acute sinusitis begins as a cold and usually resolves itself within ten days. Chronic sinusitis lasts for at least twelve weeks and may be caused by allergies, respiratory tract infections, diseases, or nasal problems. Corticosteriods or antibiotics are sometimes given to reduce inflammation and destroy the infection, if bacterial.

Gallic acid, a constituent in apple cider vinegar, has been shown to inhibit histamine and pro-inflammatory cytokines that cause inflammation of the airways and mucus production.[61] By obstructing these compounds, tissue in the airways shrink, mucus is removed, and the flow of air through the sinuses is greatly increased. At the onset of a cold, heat 1 cup of water and add 2 tablespoons of apple cider vinegar, 1 tablespoon of fresh lemon juice, and 1 tablespoon of local raw honey. Sip this drink three times a day to drain the mucus, reduce inflamed tissue, and open the airways for easier breathing. Acetic acid and the phenolic acids are all antimicrobial compounds and can destroy the spread of infection to others, whether it is bacterial, viral, or fungal. Frequent hand washing in a diluted apple cider vinegar solution as well as using this solution to clean counters, doorknobs, and stair railings will destroy the pathogens by crossing their cell membranes and disrupting metabolic functions. Others touching these surfaces will not contract the infection.

30. SWIMMER'S EAR

Water that remains in the ear after swimming can cause an infection inside the outer ear canal. The warm, moist environment is the perfect breeding ground for bacteria that are commonly found in water. They will readily invade the skin and multiply. The infection causes itching and redness, which can escalate to severe pain in and around the ear, discharge of pus, fever, and partial or complete blockage of the ear canal. To stop the infection, doctors commonly prescribe antibiotics and eardrops that contain both antibiotics and steroids. Taking over-the-counter pain medications such as ibuprofen is also recommended.

Apple cider vinegar has the ability to destroy the bacteria causing the infection and help relieve the symptoms of swimmer's ear.

NUTRITION

HEALTH

BEAUTY

HOME

It contains the anti-inflammatory compound gallic acid, which can inhibit histamine and prevent the inflammatory response. This reduces swelling and redness and allows the tissues to relieve pressure on the nerves to reduce pain. Apple cider vinegar's anti-bacterial agents can destroy the source of the infection so the ear tissues can regain their health. The acetic acid in vinegar is able to penetrate bacterial cell walls, disrupt their metabolic functions, and cause cell death. Vinegar in the treatment of swimmer's ear was found to be just as effective as topical antibiotics and steroids after one week of treatment.[62] Symptoms did last two days longer with the vinegar treatment, but those looking for a natural alternative should consider apple cider vinegar. The Seattle Children's Hospital Research Foundation suggests using one part vinegar to one part water to rinse infected ear canals. Lay on one side with the affected ear facing up. Fill the ear canal with the vinegar solution and let it remain there for five minutes. Turn the head to the side and drain the liquid. Continue this each day until the infection clears up. If the eardrum is perforated or the child has ear tubes, do not use this method.

31. URINARY TRACT INFECTIONS

Urinary tract infections involve any part of the urinary tract and include the bladder, urethra, kidneys, and ureters. Infections of the bladder are most common. Bacteria in the stool, commonly *E. coli*, can adhere to the skin and make their way into the urethra. Once there, the bacteria move up into the bladder and begin to multiply.

Initially, symptoms are not evident, but as the infection progresses, urine output changes. Many report a frequent urge to urinate, burning urination, and urine that smells bad or is cloudy, red, or pink. Pain in the pelvis or abdomen is sometimes seen, and nausea and vomiting can occur. Most urinary tract infections are treated with a course of antibiotics. Sometimes, if the pain or burning sensation is severe, doctors may prescribe pain relievers to numb the bladder and urethra.

As a preventative for urinary tract infections or for use in the early stages of an infection, drink 2 tablespoons of apple cider vinegar in 1 cup of water three times a day. This will create a slightly acidic urine environment for the infectious bacteria and discourage its growth.[63] It should be discontinued, however, if voiding is painful or if the infection is severe. The more acidic urine may further irritate the already inflamed and sensitive lining of the bladder and ureters. It is thought that the slight temporary acidity of the urine created by ingesting apple cider vinegar can work toward preventing a urinary tract infection or stopping one in its early stages.

32. VARICOSE VEINS

Varicose veins are twisted, enlarged veins near the surface of the skin. They are most common on the legs and feet because standing upright puts more pressure on the veins in the lower body. With increased pressure from gravity, the veins of the legs work harder to return blood back to the heart. Tiny valves in the veins open to allow blood to flow upward and close to prevent blood from

NUTRITION

HEALTH

BEAUTY

HOME

flowing backward toward the feet. They begin to lose elasticity and become weak. Blood starts to pool in the veins, which enlarge and become varicose. They look dark blue, swollen, and enlarged. For many, varicose veins do not pose any health problems, but if the condition is more severe, the legs may become achy, heavy, tired, swollen, or itchy. Wearing compression socks, elevating the legs, and getting exercise are good home remedies. More severe cases may opt for medical procedures to close off the veins or remove them.

Apple cider vinegar was tested alongside doctor-recommended conventional treatment on 120 patients in a randomized controlled trial. The vinegar was applied to a cloth and wrapped around the affected area of the legs for thirty minutes. This was repeated twice a day for a month. At the end of the trial, a reduction in pain and leg fatigue was higher in the group using apple cider vinegar. This same group also had a statistically significant decrease in cramps, itching, swelling, pigmentation, and feeling of heaviness in the legs.[64] It is possible that the anti-inflammatory effects of gallic acid reduced the swelling and both gallic acid and malic acid helped lower pain levels. Apple cider vinegar can also be combined with witch hazel to minimize swelling and shrink the enlarged veins. Rub over the veins for several weeks to see improvements.

MANAGING WELL-BEING

33. ACHILLES TENDONITIS

The Achilles tendon connects the calf muscle at the back of the lower leg to the heel bone. Overuse of this tendon can tear its tiny fibers. The tendon becomes swollen and painful, resulting in Achilles tendonitis. Sometimes, the sheath surrounding the tendon becomes irritated by the swollen tendon tissue underneath and it too becomes inflamed and swollen. There is little blood supply to the area, so recovery can be very slow and typically takes three to nine months. Anti-inflammatories to reduce pain and swelling are often prescribed by doctors.

Gallic acid in apple cider vinegar is an anti-inflammatory compound. It prevents inflammation and swelling, which subsequently alleviates pressure on the nerves and may be responsible for reducing pain associated with Achilles tendonitis. Acetic acid, another compound in apple cider vinegar, has proved effective in the treatment of this condition. One study used a 4 percent acetic acid solution applied through iontophoresis therapy in which the vinegar was delivered through the skin's outermost layer by electric current. Only one patient was included in the study, but it was found that pain improved after the first treatment. By the third treatment, the patient no longer needed to use a handrail with stairs, and by the fifth treatment, the patient was so improved that physical therapy was no longer needed.[65] Home treatment by soaking a cloth in apple cider vinegar and wrapping around the Achilles tendon for thirty minutes each day can be used. Repeat each day until the condition improves.

34. ADRENAL FATIGUE

Adrenal fatigue is a syndrome in which the adrenal glands are not functioning at optimal levels. These glands are responsible for producing the hormones cortisol, adrenaline, noradrenaline, and aldosterone, which are used to regulate blood pressure, sugar levels, and metabolism and to control stress. This syndrome is not a proven medical condition, but many believe that even slight decreases in adrenal hormones can affect the body, even if these levels are not detectable by medical testing. Prolonged or excessive stress is commonly associated with the onset of adrenal fatigue and can cause poor concentration and extreme tiredness.

Apple cider vinegar cannot make the adrenal glands increase their output of hormones, but it can be used to address the symptoms felt with this condition. Regulating blood sugar is very important to maintain energy levels and prevent fatigue. If the adrenal glands are not regulating their output of cortisol closely, blood sugar levels will fluctuate, and fatigue and foggy thinking can set in. Studies have uncovered apple cider vinegar as an effective agent for controlling blood sugar levels. Four random-ized crossover trials in adults found that 2 teaspoons of vinegar with a bagel and juice effectively reduced the amount of glucose in the blood by 20 percent compared to placebo.[66] These research-ers have also demonstrated an improvement in insulin sensitivity by 19 percent in type 2 diabetic patients and 34 percent in insu-lin-resistant subjects.[67] Insulin sends signals to the cells to take up glucose from the blood, normalizing blood sugar levels after a meal.

Vinegar may work by delaying the rate of gastric emptying.[68] This would slow the uptake of sugar into the blood and allow the body more time to effectively manage glucose levels. Another theory is that vinegar may prevent the complete digestion of complex carbohydrates or slow their conversion into sugar. This would mean fewer sugars are present in the blood at any one time, lessening the potential for an influx of too much glucose for the body to handle. Apple cider vinegar, then, may be valuable in controlling blood sugar levels and managing the symptoms of adrenal fatigue.

35. BAD BREATH

Bad breath is a concern for many and can be a source of em-barrassment. The shelves of pharmacies and grocery stores are filled with mints and gums to try to mask bad odors with minty or fruit-flavored products. Mouthwashes are used to attack the odor-causing bacteria in the mouth. Poor dental hygiene is a pri-mary cause for bad breath, and a more regimented and thorough mouth cleansing routine can help kill the bacteria that cause the odors. For others, however, bad breath is a result of tobacco, medications, dry mouth, infections, or disease.

An effective preventative for bad breath is to use apple cider vinegar as a mouthwash just before brushing. The acids in the vinegar are antibacterial and will eliminate bacteria in the mouth by crossing their cell membranes and disrupting metabolic functions, causing cell death. Add 1 tablespoon to 1/2 cup of water and swirl around the mouth for thirty seconds. Apple cider vinegar is very acidic and can erode the tooth's enamel. For this reason, never use it undiluted and follow by brushing with toothpaste or baking soda. This is a safe and inexpensive way to improve any oral hygiene routine for the prevention and treatment of bad breath.

36. BONE SPURS

Cartilage can get worn down from osteoarthritis, causing a loss of cushioning between the joints. The body tries to compensate for this loss by depositing calcium, which causes a bony protrusion, or bone spur, near the damaged area. These bony projections occur along the edges of bones and are most common in the knees, spine, fingers, shoulders, hips, and heels. The spurs themselves are painless, but the soft tissue around them becomes inflamed, which can cause acute or chronic pain throughout the day. In most cases, over-the-counter pain relievers are used to reduce the inflamed tissue and any pain. If the bone spurs are limiting movement or pressing on nerves causing numbness or severe pain, surgery may be needed to remove them.

The acetic acid in apple cider vinegar has been proven to be an effective treatment for bone spurs in the heel. Thirty-five patients with chronic heel pain were treated over a four-year period with acetic acid iontophoresis. This process uses a low electric current to send acetic acid through the outermost layers of skin. An astounding 94 percent of patients had total or substantial relief in heel pain from six or fewer sessions in under three weeks. After two years, heel pain had not returned.[69] Another study used acetic acid iontophoresis in patients with plantar fasciitis, which is often a cause of bone spurs in heels. They demonstrated that acetic acid relieved patient pain as well as the steroid medication dexamethasone.[70] It is thought that the vinegar works by combining its acetic acid with the calcium carbonate of the bone spurs. This forms calcium acetate, which dissolves in the blood. The bone spur is washed away over time. Iontophoresis cannot be used at home, but applying apple cider vinegar topically to the site of the bone spur can allow the vinegar to penetrate at its own rate and take action.

37. BURNS

A burn damages the skin and possibly underlying tissues and can be caused by sunlight, heat, chemicals, electricity, or radiation. There are three types of burns: First-degree burns affect the outer layer of skin and cause minor inflammation, redness, and pain. Second-degree burns damage the outer layer of skin and the layer underneath. They are characterized by blisters, redness, and pain. Third-degree burns are the most serious and damage the deepest layer of skin tissue. They have a white, leathery appearance.

NUTRITION

HEALTH

BEAUTY

HOME

Treatment for minor burns includes cleaning the wound, applying antibiotic cream, and taking pain medication. More severe burns should be treated by a medical professional.

Apple cider vinegar can be used in the treatment of minor burns. This is a ready and inexpensive remedy that can be prepared at home. The gallic acid in apple cider vinegar has been found to reduce local inflammation by blocking the release of histamine and pro-inflammatory cytokines. It helps reduce swelling of the burned tissue and decreases redness and pain. The acids in apple cider vinegar are also antibacterial and can attack any bacteria around the damaged skin. This discourages infection and helps the immune system to heal the burn. After cooling down the skin with water, apply a cloth soaked in a solution of 1 cup apple cider vinegar and 1 cup water. Wrap around the burn for fifteen minutes. Repeat as necessary.

38. BURSITIS

The lubricating fluid between tissues like bones, tendons, muscles, and skin decreases friction and rubbing between tissues and allows for easy, comfortable movement. Bursa are fluid-filled sacs that decrease friction between bones, tendons, and muscles. They are found typically around joints such as the knee, hip, and shoulder. When these sacs of fluid become inflamed, the painful condition that results is bursitis. Whether it be from injury or overuse, bursitis is caused when protein from the bursa or surrounding tissue is broken down, creating a slightly alkaline environment in that area. Calcium is then deposited in the bursa because of the rise in pH, causing inflammation, redness, and pain. Bursitis should go away within a week, but if it doesn't, corticosteroids can be given to reduce inflammation and bring rapid pain relief.

There are many home remedies that use between 1 and 2 tablespoons of apple cider vinegar a day to treat bursitis. The anti-inflammatory properties of gallic acid in the vinegar can reduce swelling and redness in the bursa by inhibiting the release of histamines and pro-inflammatory cytokines so that the immune system does not initiate the inflammatory response. When tissue swelling is reduced, the pressure on surrounding nerves is decreased and they no longer send pain signals. As part of the healing process, the calcium deposits need to be removed from the bursa. The alkaline environment created in the bursa by the breakdown of protein causes calcium to be precipitated in the tissue. Some believe that drinking apple cider vinegar will alter the pH of the bursa tissue into a slightly acidic environment for a period so the calcium can dissolve and be removed. While the exact mechanism by which apple cider vinegar works has not been thoroughly investigated, many attest to its effectiveness. It should be noted that there is no scientific evidence supporting the theory that foods can alter the pH level of the body. Acidic foods can increase the acidity of urine, but the body tightly regulates body pH regardless of the foods eaten.

As mentioned, incorporating apple cider vinegar into the diet can provide these benefits for bursitis, but if the taste is off-putting, try soaking a cloth in a warm solution of one part vinegar and one part water and wrap the area. Cover with a towel and let sit for thirty minutes. Repeat as needed for relief.

NUTRITION

HEALTH

BEAUTY

HOME

39. CHRONIC FATIGUE

This syndrome is characterized by extreme fatigue that is not relieved by rest. It is accompanied by headaches, muscle pain, joint pain, sleep problems, tender lymph nodes, or memory loss. It is not known what causes chronic fatigue, but hormonal imbalances, some viral infections, or impaired immune systems may be triggers. Restrictions in daily activity are common, and those with chronic fatigue often feel depressed. To aid with the symptoms, antidepressants are frequently taken to help with mood, pain, and sleep.

Malic acid is a constituent of apple cider vinegar that is commonly known to increase energy and reduce pain. The University of Maryland Medical Center suggests that magnesium combined with malic acid can reduce fatigue and boost energy. Together, they metabolize carbohydrates and increase energy in the body. A reduction in fatigue as well as pain should be noticeable after a few days. Scientists have found that patients using a combination of malic acid and magnesium reported improvements in pain and stiffness[71, 72] and had a more positive outlook. Taking an apple cider vinegar supplement along with a magnesium supplement may provide these benefits. To get them from food, try making a smoothie that includes a banana, some spinach, and 2 tablespoons of apple cider vinegar. Apple cider vinegar also increases iron absorption.[73] This is needed in the body to deliver oxygen to cells and is used to enhance energy, mood, and concentration.

40. CLEAN WOUNDS

Wounding the skin is a very common occurrence and happens to everyone. Whether it's slicing the tip of a finger while dicing carrots or slipping on gravel and scraping a knee, cuts and scrapes tear the skin tissue and often cause bleeding. If the wound is deep, bleeds heavily, or has an object embedded in it, seek medical attention. If it's minor, however, it can be addressed at home. Wash your hands with soap and water. Clean the wound by pouring cool, clean water over it to remove dirt and debris. Then wash with soap and water. Once clean, an antibiotic ointment can be applied.

Here is where apple cider vinegar comes in. Apple cider vinegar is an antibacterial, antiviral, and antifungal agent that can attack and kill many pathogens that find their way into an open wound. This discourages infection and helps the immune system heal the skin. Sometimes, there is pain and swelling in and around the wound. Apple cider vinegar reduces these symptoms by lowering histamine and pro-inflammatory cytokines.[74] This prevents inflammation of the tissue around the wound and reduces itching and redness. Pressure on the nerves from the swollen tissue eases, and pain is reduced. Apple cider vinegar can be diluted with a little bit of water or applied directly to the skin around the wound to prevent infection and begin the healing process.

NUTRITION

HEALTH

BEAUTY

HOME

41. COLDS

Common colds are respiratory illnesses caused by viruses. They are highly contagious, and a person can become infected by touching a surface such as a doorknob, stair railing, or bathroom faucet. If the virus gets on the hands and the person then touches their mouth or nose, the virus nestles into the mucosal lining there. Breathing in air near someone who is coughing or sneezing because they are sick with a cold is another surefire way of getting the virus into the system. There are many different viruses that cause colds. Unless the body has fought the exact virus before, it won't have the right antibodies ready to fight it when it enters the body. The immune system begins an attack against the new virus, and the dreaded symptoms set in. A sore throat, runny or stuffy nose, sneezing, and coughing are the hallmarks of a cold. There is no shortage of over-the-counter cold medications, and they are available for every possible symptom. Take a walk down the pharmacy aisle to see antihistamines, decongestants, nasal sprays, cough suppressants, and throat lozenges.

An inexpensive and effective home remedy to combat these symptoms is to use apple cider vinegar. In fact, Hippocrates was said to have recommended mixing apple cider vinegar with honey for the treatment of colds as long ago as 400 BC. It is a known antiviral and can help the body get rid of the virus. It provides support to the immune system and will shorten the duration of the illness. Gallic acid in apple cider vinegar can also reduce the symptoms caused by the virus. It has been shown to inhibit histamine and pro-inflammatory cytokines that cause inflammation of the sinuses and mucus production.[75] These compounds trigger reactions that make noses stuffy and chests congested. By obstructing these compounds, tissue in the sinuses shrink, mucus is removed, and the flow of air is greatly increased. This allows for a restful night's sleep to reduce fatigue and give the body time and energy to conquer the virus. Take 2 tablespoons in a glass of water three times a day.

42. CONSTIPATION

Constipation is infrequent bowel movements or difficulty in passing stools. It is very common and can be occasional or chronic. Occasional constipation is short term, while chronic constipation is having less than three bowel movements a week for at least three months. Stools move too slowly through the digestive tract and become hard and dry. They are difficult to pass, and a feeling of not being able to empty the rectum is reported. Increasing fiber intake, fluids, and exercise are known to help increase gastric motility. If that doesn't work, laxatives and other medications to draw water into the intestines are suggested. Side effects of these drugs include bloating, gas, diarrhea, nausea, vomiting, and rectal pain.

Apple cider vinegar can be used for gastrointestinal support. This is significant for those suffering from constipation who want a natural way to stimulate their system. Chlorogenic acid in apple cider vinegar is a natural laxative and can induce muscle contractions in the colon. These contractions force waste to move through the intestinal system and out of the body, relieving constipation. Vinegar may also prevent the complete digestion of complex carbohydrates or slow their conversion into sugar. This makes these carbohydrates available to feed the good bacteria in the intestines. A healthy supply of good bacteria is essential to make vitamins, improve digestion, boost immunity, and relieve gastrointestinal distress. For constipation, take 2 tablespoons of apple cider vinegar in a glass of water three times a day. It is not only the vinegar but also the increased fluid intake with the water that will help move the stool through the system.

43. DEPRESSION

Depression is a mood disorder that causes a deep sadness and a loss of interest in activities. It affects how a person feels, thinks, and behaves and can cause not just emotional problems but physical problems as well. Clinical depression many occur once in a person's lifetime or reoccur multiple times. This feeling of sadness and loss can cause insomnia, loss of appetite, poor concentration, fatigue, suicidal thoughts, and physical symptoms like backaches and headaches. Changes in the body's hormone levels may cause or trigger depression. Modifications to the way brain chemicals work and the effect that has on maintaining stable moods is thought to play a major role in depression. Psychological counseling and antidepressant medications are often prescribed. Antidepressants can cause a wide range of side effects, including nausea, insomnia, blurred vision, weight gain, fatigue, and sexual dysfunction.

Apple cider vinegar can play a role in mental health. A pilot study on older healthy adults found that chlorogenic acid (as found in apple cider vinegar) is capable of improving mood.[76] Another role is through its other acids. Consuming apple cider vinegar may help increase the availability of raw materials needed for the production of "feel good" hormones by temporarily increasing stomach acid. Because many people have low stomach acid, supplementing with an external source can increase the digestion of protein. Low stomach acid does not digest protein properly, which then enters the small intestine and puts stress on the pancreas to finish the process. The pancreas can get worn out, and protein breakdown and absorption decreases further. Vital protein is lost through elimination and not available for the production of hormones and neurotransmitters like serotonin, dopamine, and oxytocin. Apple cider vinegar can assist in driving the process that forms these chemicals, which can lift mood and bring on feelings of happiness and satisfaction.

44. DIARRHEA

Diarrhea describes loose, watery stools. It is very common and usually lasts a few days, although prolonged diarrhea can indicate a medical condition like irritable bowel syndrome. Stomach cramps and pain, bloating, fever, nausea, and vomiting often accompany diarrhea. It occurs when the stool moves too quickly through the colon so that the colon doesn't have time to absorb enough liquid from it. The main culprits in causing diarrhea are viruses, bacteria, and parasites. Food intolerance and many medications can also cause diarrhea in susceptible people. If diarrhea persists for more than a few days, doctors may prescribe antibiotics if the cause is bacterial or parasitic.

Apple cider vinegar has the power to destroy germs in the intestinal system responsible for causing diarrhea. Acetic acid and phenolic acids have antibiotic properties and can be used to combat intestinal infections by inhibiting the proliferation of bacteria. These acids are able to cross the bacterial cell membranes and disrupt metabolic functions, causing cell death. If diarrhea is virally induced, apple cider vinegar's antiviral compounds can attack and destroy the viral infection and alleviate the condition. Sometimes, diarrhea is caused by rapid gastric emptying, which is common after abdominal surgery and in those with diabetes. Apple cider vinegar slows the rate of gastric emptying,[77] which allows the intestinal system more time to remove water from the waste before it leaves the body. The stool becomes firmer and can pass normally. Apple cider vinegar can be used as an effective and natural alternative to relieve diarrhea with little to no side effects.

Apple cider vinegar that is ingested gets rapidly absorbed in the gastrointestinal system and broken down. In order for the acetic and phenolic acids to work on the pathogens causing diarrhea, they have to reach the bacteria in the intestines intact. Consuming apple cider vinegar in an enteric-coated capsule would deliver this. Then they can work directly on the bacteria and destroy them.

45. DIZZINESS

Dizziness is a term that is used to describe feelings of being lightheaded, faint, or weak. It may or may not involve nausea, vomiting, or vertigo—a sensation that surroundings are moving when there is no actual movement. Most people experience harmless episodes of dizziness now and again, which are usually caused by inner ear disturbances or motion sickness, in which signals received from the eyes, the body, and the inner ear send conflicting messages to the brain. Frequent or severe dizziness may have an underlying medical cause such as injury, infection, or poor circulation. Dizziness usually goes away on its own, but if it is impairing quality of life, a number of medications exist for its treatment, including antinausea drugs, antianxiety drugs, antihistamine drugs, or water pills.

Adding apple cider vinegar into the diet can better control dizziness related to blood sugar levels. Four randomized crossover trials in adults given 2 teaspoons of vinegar with a meal showed that the amount of glucose in the blood was reduced by 20 percent compared to placebo.[78] These researchers also demonstrated a 19 to 34 percent improvement in insulin sensitivity in their subjects.[79] Insulin that works better to encourage glucose uptake from the blood into the cells can help manage blood sugar levels and reduce the effects of any dizziness that may result.

Vinegar may work by delaying the rate of gastric emptying.[80] This would slow the uptake of sugar into the blood and allow the body more time to effectively manage glucose levels. Another theory is that vinegar may prevent the complete digestion of complex carbohydrates or slow their conversion into sugar. This would mean fewer sugars are present in the blood at any one time, lessening the potential for an influx of too much glucose for the body to handle.

NUTRITION

HEALTH

BEAUTY

HOME

46. ENERGY LAPSES

Everyone has lulls of energy in their day that have them longing for a quick catnap on the couch. They often reach for caffeinated beverages to boost their energy and awaken their minds. A combination of factors can lead to low energy, and common ones are lack of sleep, poor diet, stress, and depression. Taking care to manage the source that drains energy would be a good first step to give bodies what they need to function properly and provide enough energy to happily get through the day. Going to bed earlier, cutting back on saturated fats and sugar, finding outlets to deal with stress, or talking to a therapist are all ways to do this. However, to add even more pep to your step, try taking a little apple cider vinegar every day.

Malic acid and acetic acid found in apple cider vinegar both enhance iron absorption.[81] This is good news, since iron is commonly deficient in the diet. Iron functions primarily in the formation of hemoglobin, an essential molecule that carries oxygen in red blood cells to all the tissues of the body. Without this oxygen, these tissues would not be able to survive. Similarly, iron is a key component of myoglobin, which also holds oxygen and carries it to the skeletal muscles and heart. Oxygen raises energy levels by burning glucose.

If iron is not available in sufficient amounts in the body, oxygen is not delivered to the tissues and both mental and physical fatigue set in. The acids in apple cider vinegar can be used to increase the amount of iron from food through the digestive process to give the body the oxygen necessary to stimulate the mind and energize the body. To take advantage of the iron in your food, take 1 to 2 tablespoons of apple cider vinegar in 1 cup of water before each meal.

47. EXERCISE-INDUCED MUSCLE PAIN

After months of inactivity, going out for a competitive game of flag football or a vigorous evening run with a friend may seem like a good idea. However, trying to move about the next day when every muscle is stiff and sore will squelch that belief. Taking preventative measures to guard against injury-induced muscle pain or aches from overuse are something to think about for next time. Muscle aches can also result from tension, stress, or disease. The pain can be anywhere in the body and can last from several hours to months. If exercise induced, muscle pain results from microscopic tears in the muscle fibers; if disease related, muscle pain can be caused by inflammation.

Apple cider vinegar has proven effective in treating muscle damage after moderate intensity exercise. In a double-blind placebo-controlled crossover trial, forty participants were supplemented with acetic acid bacteria or cornstarch. Acetic acid bacteria is what is found in the Mother of raw apple cider vinegar and is used in the fermentation process to create vinegar. At the end of the study, it was found that creatine kinase was significantly lower in the acetic acid bacteria supplement group. This is an enzyme that is commonly found in damaged skeletal muscles, which means less damage was produced in the muscles of the participants in the group supplemented with acetic acid bacteria. Ankle pain was also significantly lower, as were neutrophil counts, which are involved in inflammation. Malic acid in apple cider vinegar can also reduce muscle pain and tenderness when combined with magnesium.[82] Taking apple cider vinegar before exercise reduces muscle damage, inflammation, and pain. Make sure to use a brand that contains the Mother to provide the benefits of the acetic acid bacteria.

48. HEADACHES AND MIGRAINES

A headache is a pain in any part of the head and may be sharp, dull, or throbbing. It can last from under an hour to several days. Migraines are severe headaches that cause intense pain, usually on one side of the head, and are accompanied by nausea, vomiting, and sensitivity to light and sound. Migraines can come with warning signs such as blind spots in the field of vision, flashes of light, or tingling sensations on the face, arms, or legs. Migraines can be so severe that the person can't function normally and often requires rest and isolation to recover. Causes of migraines are different for everyone. Some triggers could be changes in hormone levels, food allergies, stress, some medications, sensory stimuli, or changes in the environment, like a fall in barometric pressure from an approaching storm. Regular headaches can be caused by a multitude of factors, from dehydration to too little sleep to infections. They may also be symptoms of disease. Pain-relieving medications are commonly used to deal with the symptoms. In the case of migraines, antinausea medications are also prescribed.

Apple cider vinegar contains an anti-inflammatory substance called gallic acid. This can provide headache and migraine relief by inhibiting histamine and pro-inflammatory cytokines that cause inflammation and subsequent pain from compressed nerves. Gallic acid is also an astringent and can shrink the blood vessels that become dilated and cause throbbing pain. Next time a headache appears, try consuming between 1 teaspoon and 1 tablespoon of apple cider vinegar in 1 cup of water as well as soaking a cotton ball in apple cider vinegar and applying the liquid directly to the affected area of the head. Another method is inhaling the steam of equal parts apple cider vinegar and water for a minute as it heats on the stove.

49. HEAD LICE

Every year, it seems children are sent home from school with a note warning parents that there is an outbreak of head lice in the school. These tiny insects that infest children's (and adults'!) scalps are a source of panic and embarrassment, although having lice is not a sign of poor personal hygiene. They can fall off the head and land on carpet, bedding, towels, and stuffed animals, where they can lay their eggs and continue to grow for another day or two. Lice feed on the blood of the scalp and are readily transferred from one person to another through direct contact. A person may be infected for several weeks before itching begins. The itching is an allergic reaction to the louse saliva. The lice and nits (eggs) are difficult to see, but a close look around the ears and neckline may provide the best chance of glimpsing them. Over-the-counter and prescription medicated shampoos are used to kill the adult lice. The eggs are hard to get rid of because they adhere to the hair shaft with a sticky substance that is difficult to wash out. A second treatment of medicated shampoo is recommended when the nits hatch.

The acetic acid in apple cider vinegar can be used to loosen the sticky glue-like substance that holds the nits to the hair. They can then be easily removed with a fine-tooth comb. The vinegar is very safe to use on the scalp and has the added benefits of removing product buildup on the hair and boosting shine. Apple cider vinegar is an excellent complement to medicated shampoos, and the end result will be the removal of all stages of the lice life cycle in one day rather than having to wait seven to nine days for retreatment.

50. HEARTBURN/ACID REFLUX

Heartburn is also known as acid reflux. It occurs when acid splashes up into the esophagus from the stomach and causes a burning pain in the chest. Those who suffer from heartburn will notice that it is often worse after eating and at night. The acid travels more easily up the esophagus when bending over or lying down. Most people tend to think that heartburn is caused by too much stomach acid, but actually the opposite is much more common. Low stomach acid means the stomach must work harder to try to break down food. It churns more vigorously and can cause some of the acid to splash up. If the valve separating the esophagus from the stomach is weakened, the acid will enter the esophagus and cause the burning sensation of heartburn. Over-the-counter medications are taken to reduce or neutralize the stomach acid. These can cause nausea, constipation, diarrhea, headache, and abdominal pain. Some of these seem worse than the heartburn itself.

Apple cider vinegar is widely used as a natural remedy for the treatment of heartburn without the side effects of commonly used medications. The acetic acid in the vinegar increases the amount of acid in the stomach, which helps digest food. Because it is a weaker acid than the hydrochloric acid in the stomach, a milder acidic environment is temporarily maintained for digestion. This is still sufficient for efficient digestion, and the stomach no longer has to churn as forcefully to try to digest food with limited acid. In addition, if any acid does splash up, it won't be as acidic and therefore not as harsh on the esophagus. Taking 2 to 3 teaspoons in a glass of water about five minutes before a meal should help prevent heartburn.

51. HEMORRHOIDS

Hemorrhoids are swollen veins in the rectum and anus. The walls of the veins can stretch and cause the blood vessels to bulge. Internal hemorrhoids are inside the rectum and can bleed into the stool. This area has few pain receptors, so hemorrhoids here generally do not hurt. External hemorrhoids are located on the anus where there are more pain-sensing nerves. These can be quite sore, especially during a bowel movement. They develop from a buildup of pressure in the lower rectum that can affect the flow of blood and cause the veins to swell. Straining during a bowel movement, pregnancy, or obesity can cause them. Hemorrhoids are extremely common and can cause bleeding, itching, pain, and inflammation. Topical creams or suppositories, cold packs, and oral pain relievers can help symptoms subside.

Swiping a cotton ball dipped in apple cider vinegar directly over the affected area can alleviate the symptoms of hemorrhoids. Let the area air dry and reapply as necessary. The astringent properties of gallic acid, found in apple cider vinegar, will shrink the blood vessel tissue, decreasing the size of the hemorrhoid and relieving pressure. Bleeding will be reduced, and bowel movements become more comfortable. Gallic acid also inhibits inflammatory compounds from inducing swelling and itching. The end result is shrunken hemorrhoid tissue, decreased bleeding, and alleviation of pain and itching.

52. HICCUPS

Hiccups are involuntary reflex contractions of the diaphragm, the muscle separating the chest from the abdomen. A quarter of a second after the diaphragm contracts, the vocal cords snap shut and cause the characteristic "hic" sound for which the condition is named. A single hiccup or a series of hiccups may start suddenly and often subside on their own within a few minutes. Swallowing too much air, excitement or stress, laughing, coughing, or some medical conditions like acid reflux or diabetes can trigger them. If hiccups persist for longer than two days, several medications can be prescribed that act to relax muscles, prevent spasms, or reduce acid reflux.

Hiccups can be incredibly annoying and disruptive. Everyone has an opinion on how to get rid of them, but there is no consensus on what actually works. Many people have used apple cider vinegar with success. A possible explanation could be that the acid in the vinegar irritates the pharynx, which aggravates the vagus nerve—part of the hiccup reflex control center. Overstimulating the vagus nerve might block signals to the vocal cords during an episode of hiccups and return them to normal function. If acid reflux is the trigger for hiccups, apple cider vinegar can calm the stomach from churning up acid and splashing it into the esophagus. Just drink 1 teaspoon of apple cider vinegar in 1/2 cup of water at the onset of hiccups to experience immediate relief.

53. HOT FLASHES

When women enter their menopausal years, up to two-thirds of them experience hot flashes, the sudden onset of intense heat or warmth in the face, neck, and chest. They can be accompanied by rapid heartbeat, flushed red skin, and sweating. Each woman's experience is different. Some have them for only a short period of time, while others continue to get them throughout their lives. Whether it happens a few times a day or several times an hour, the severity of hot flashes tends to decrease over time. Around the time of menopause, a woman's reproductive hormone balance changes and the hypothalamus, which regulates the body temperature, may also be experiencing some changes. It is thought that these two may play a role in the onset of hot flashes. When the body temperature rises, the blood vessels near the surface of the skin

NUTRITION
HEALTH
BEAUTY
HOME

NUTRITION

HEALTH

BEAUTY

HOME

dilate in an attempt to cool the body down. Women may opt to take hormones to prevent hot flashes if they are severe or interfere with daily life. Estrogen or a combination of estrogen and progesterone are commonly prescribed. Antidepressants and antiseizure medications are also given to reduce hot flashes. These drugs can increase the risk of breast cancer, stroke, heart disease, and blood clots. They can also cause irritability, anxiety, nausea, and fatigue. These are just some of the side effects.

There are many testimonials on the effectiveness of apple cider vinegar in the treatment of hot flashes. While there is no medical evidence to suggest it works, the lack of data simply means it hasn't been tested in a controlled study. The fact that many women swear by it means that it is a probable alternative treatment to medical drugs. At the very least, drinking apple cider vinegar provides a safe and natural option with other health benefits, including increased weight loss and decreased high blood pressure. According to the Mayo Clinic, a high body mass index in women is associated with a higher frequency of hot flashes. Lowering weight may help reduce the incidence or severity of hot flashes in these women. Women experiencing hot flashes also have higher systolic blood pressure.[83] Acetic acid, the main component of apple cider vinegar, was found to significantly reduce blood pressure by decreasing compounds that constrict the arteries and increase blood volume, both of which lead to higher blood pressure.[84] It also contains chlorogenic acid, which was proven to reduce blood pressure in mildly hypertensive people without any side effects.[85] Women have reported taking anywhere from 2 teaspoons of apple cider vinegar to 6 tablespoons in divided doses each day. It would be advisable to begin with a smaller amount and gradually increase the dose until you experience improvement. The vinegar can be diluted in water, apple juice, tea, or a drink sweetened with honey, maple syrup, or stevia.

54. HPV DETECTION

HPV stands for human papillomavirus, and there are over one hundred varieties that exist. Most commonly, it causes growths on the skin and mucous membranes and is responsible for common warts, plantar warts, and genital warts. Other types can cause cervical or other types of genital cancers. Many times, the virus goes away on its own. Genital warts and cancers can develop in some, particularly in those with compromised immune systems. The virus is contagious and enters the skin through cuts or abrasions. Topical medications or surgical procedures can remove warts, but cancers are often treated with radiation, chemotherapy, and surgery.

It is interesting to note that apple cider vinegar can be used to treat HPV that causes common and plantar warts. The phenolic acids and acetic acid in the vinegar have antiviral properties and are able to destroy HPV after several applications. Acetic acid in apple cider vinegar is also used to diagnose HPV infections in the genital area. Sometimes, the lesions are flat and difficult to see. Washing the area with acetic acid turns the lesions white with clear borders, enabling the doctor to identify them and treat them on site. These vinegar washes are also used by midwives in remote areas like Peru and Zimbabwe to screen women for HPV infection.[86] In fact, the vinegar washes are sensitive enough to rapidly detect about 77 percent of abnormal tissue, about the same rate as achieved with Pap smears.[87]

55. INCREASE MINERAL ABSORPTION

Minerals make up about 5 percent of our body weight, mostly in the skeleton. Macrominerals like calcium, magnesium, and phosphorus are needed in larger quantities than microminerals like iron, but all are equally vital for good health. They are so important that vitamins cannot carry out their jobs properly without them. The only way to get minerals is from the earth, through intake of food and water. When the body is unable to absorb enough nutrients, a mineral deficiency occurs. This can happen gradually.

Calcium is the most abundant mineral in our bodies. It is best known for its role in the development and maintenance of healthy teeth and bones. As people get older—particularly women—ensuring adequate levels of calcium intake is extremely important to prevent osteoporosis. It plays an important part in the cardiovascular system by helping maintain a regular heartbeat, reducing cholesterol, assisting in blood clotting, and potentially lowering blood pressure. Calcium is also known to help prevent cancer and is useful in keeping the skin looking healthy. Inadequate calcium levels can lead to osteoporosis, brittle nails, irregular heartbeat, muscle cramps, and insomnia.

Considered the "antistress" mineral, magnesium is a natural tranquilizer that relaxes the skeletal muscles and the smooth muscles of blood vessels and the gastrointestinal tract. It's important to the cardiovascular system because it can prevent heart attacks, lower blood cholesterol, and decrease hypertension (high blood pressure). Research shows magnesium also helps play a role in preventing osteoporosis and certain forms of cancer as well as helping to alleviate the symptoms of premenstrual syndrome. Experiencing muscle spasms, gallstones, irregular heartbeat, excessive body odor, or cravings for chocolate may indicate a magnesium deficiency.

Most phosphorus is deposited in the bones, with a bit in the teeth and the rest in other cells of the body. It is involved in the formation of bones and teeth, cell growth, blood clotting, and kidney function. It's important to have enough phosphorus to help keep a normal heart rhythm and strong contractions of the heart. Too much, however, can compete with calcium for absorption in the intestines and cause an imbalance in the ratio of phosphorus to calcium. If less calcium is available, problems with bone health can result. Another major role of phosphorus is in the conversion of food to energy. Deficiencies can cause fatigue, bone pain, irregular breathing, numbness, trembling, and anxiety. Our North American diet often provides too much phosphorus, so deficiencies are rare unless the body cannot absorb it in adequate amounts from food.

Iron functions primarily in the formation of hemoglobin, an essential molecule that carries oxygen in red blood cells to all the tissues of the body. Without this oxygen, these tissues would not be able to survive. Similarly, iron is a key component of myoglobin, which also holds oxygen and carries it to the skeletal muscles and heart. Sufficient amounts of these molecules give the body the energy for muscle performance. Unfortunately, iron is commonly deficient in the diet. Symptoms of this can include a lack of energy, pale lower eyelids, dizziness, a rapid heart rate, a craving for ice, and spoon-shaped nails.

NUTRITION

HEALTH

BEAUTY

HOME

Apple cider vinegar itself doesn't contain minerals at any significant levels, but the acids in the vinegar help increase the absorption of calcium, magnesium, phosphorus, and iron from food. A study in male rats found that when acetic acids levels were increased in the waste products in the cecum of the large intestine, calcium, magnesium, and phosphorus absorption and retention were significantly elevated.[88] Another study showed that acetic acid and malic acid, found in apple cider vinegar, both enhance iron absorption in a human cell line.[89] Whether it's correcting a mineral deficiency or just getting the most nutrition out of food, consuming apple cider vinegar with meals can help increase mineral availability to the body.

56. INSECT BITES

In spring and early summer, bug bites can make sitting outside intolerable. Wearing bug repellent and long sleeves and pants or staying inside can reduce or prevent the incidence of bites, but these precautions are not infallible. Once bitten, the skin can swell, turn red, sting, and be itchy. The insects break the skin to reach the blood that they need for nourishment and to develop their eggs. Many secrete anticoagulants in their saliva to keep the blood flowing while they are trying to get a meal. The body reacts to these compounds by releasing histamines to combat the foreign substance. The blood vessels expand and irritate the nerves, causing the characteristic red, swollen, itchy bump.

Most reactions are minor and disappear in a day or two. The itching, however, can be very uncomfortable and disrupt daily living and sleep. Apply apple cider vinegar to a cotton ball and gently swipe over the irritated skin. The gallic acid in the vinegar will prevent the release of histamine from the mast cells of the immune system so that all subsequent processes of the inflammatory response will subside. Itching will disappear along with the redness and swelling. Because gallic acid is also an astringent, it can shrink blood vessel tissue, which further acts to reduce itching. Immediate relief should be experienced. Reapply apple cider vinegar as needed until itching stops altogether.

57. JELLYFISH STING

Jellyfish have long tentacles trailing from their bodies that have tiny stingers containing venom. Brushing up against a tentacle triggers the release of the tiny stingers that then penetrate the skin and inject venom. Usually, only the immediate area is affected, but if the venom enters the bloodstream, a more serious reaction can occur. Beware that jellyfish washed up on beaches are still poisonous. Even tentacles floating unattached in the water can discharge venom. There are many types of jellyfish, and most are harmless to humans. A sting will typically cause only localized pain, burning, itching, swelling, and redness.

If stung, wash the area with seawater, then remove the tentacles (don't touch them). Rinse the area liberally with vinegar for thirty seconds to deactivate the stinging cells.[90] The acids in apple cider vinegar break down proteins in the venom and neutralize it. Then soak the skin in hot water for twenty minutes. The itching can be alleviated by the presence of gallic acid in apple cider vinegar, an anti-inflammatory and astringent. Gallic acid prevents the release of histamine from the mast cells of the immune system so that the inflammatory response subsides. Itching disappears along with the redness and swelling. It also works by shrinking blood vessel tissue, stopping nerve irritation and the itch sensation. This remedy is so effective, it is practiced in coastal settings worldwide.

58. LOW STOMACH ACID

Hydrochloric acid in the stomach is needed to begin breaking down protein in food. It also stimulates the secretion of pepsin, an enzyme that further digests protein. Low levels of stomach acid are very common, particularly in older adults. With insufficient amounts of stomach acid, proteins cannot be digested properly, and vitamin B12 as well as multiple minerals and cannot be adequately absorbed. This leads to nutrient deficiencies and malnutrition, food sensitivities, increased risk of infections, and colon toxicity. Oftentimes, people with acid reflux believe they have too much stomach acid, but in reality, it is more likely to be the opposite. Not only does low stomach acid cause acid reflux, it can also cause a range of gastrointestinal upsets as well as bad breath, acne, and weak fingernails.

The way to remedy the situation is to increase the amount of acid in the stomach. Ingesting a small glass of water with 1 teaspoon of apple cider vinegar fifteen minutes before a meal will increase the amount of acid in the stomach. Don't dilute the vinegar too much, because the water will decrease the acidity in the stomach. If 1 teaspoon is not sufficient to reduce symptoms, try adding another teaspoon at the next meal. Continue this until an effective dose is found, but do not exceed 2 tablespoons per meal. The acids in the vinegar combine with hydrochloric acid to improve digestion and the assimilation of nutrients.

59. MENORRHAGIA (HEAVY MENSTRUAL FLOW)

Abnormally heavy or prolonged bleeding with menstrual periods is called menorrhagia. It is defined as bleeding heavily enough to soak one tampon or pad every hour for several consecutive hours or bleeding for more than seven days. Cramping or the passing of large blood clots can accompany blood loss. The condition can interfere with sleep or daily activities and can even be severe enough to cause anemia. There are many reasons why women experience heavy menstrual flows; hormonal imbalance, fibroids, intrauterine devices, medications, bleeding disorders, or medical conditions like polycystic ovary syndrome are some of the causes. Anti-inflammatory or blood-clotting drugs can be given to reduce blood flow and help with the pain, hormonal therapy can help rebalance the hormones, or surgery to remove uterine masses or tissue may be advised. Iron supplements are also given if the woman becomes anemic.

Gallic acid in apple cider vinegar is used internally as a remote astringent to constrict uterine tissues and stop bleeding. Taking 2 or 3 teaspoons in a glass of water every morning during menstruation should help reduce heavy bleeding. Vinegar can be used to increase insulin sensitivity. This is important if heavy bleeding is caused by polycystic ovary syndrome. If a woman has insulin resistance, her pancreas secretes more insulin to get glucose into the cells. The excess insulin can affect the ovaries' ability to ovulate by increasing androgen production. This leads to heavy bleeding. Vinegar can improve insulin sensitivity by 19 percent in type 2 diabetic patients and 34 percent in insulin-resistant subjects.[91] Apple cider vinegar can also decrease the risk of anemia through its ability to increase iron absorption, making a greater supply available to the body. If iron is not available in sufficient amounts, oxygen is not delivered to the tissues and both mental and physical fatigue set in. Apple cider vinegar, then, can give women back their energy during periods of heavy menstrual flow and allow them to continue enjoying their daily lives.

60. MENTAL FUNCTION

The ability of the brain to process thoughts, learn new information, comprehend situations, provide speech, and remember data constitutes mental function. With age, these functions can decrease. Certain medical conditions or diseases like multiple sclerosis can change neural pathways that reduce cognitive capacity.

Acetic acid bacteria found in the Mother of raw apple cider vinegar is used in the fermentation process to create vinegar. It contains sphingolipids, which are important components of brain tissue. A double-blind experiment was conducted over twelve weeks to test the continuous ingestion of acetic acid bacteria on healthy middle-aged and elderly adults. Supplementation significantly shortened response times of working memory without any side effects.[92] Consuming raw apple cider vinegar with the Mother on a daily basis can improve mental functioning and possibly prevent a decline in cognitive health with age.

61. MUSCLE CRAMPS

Muscles that suddenly contract involuntarily and become hard and painful constitute muscle cramps. The muscles most susceptible to these are the feet, calves, thighs, hands, arms, abdomen, and muscles along the sides of the ribs. There are many factors that can cause muscle cramps, but the common ones include overexertion of muscles during exercise, poor circulation, mineral depletion, or dehydration. Muscle cramps are generally harmless, and gentle stretching of the muscle that is in spasm will often release the cramp.

Deficiencies in calcium and magnesium can account for the sudden onset of some muscle cramps. Magnesium transports calcium across cell membranes, where it plays a substantial role in nerve impulse conduction and muscle contractions. In order for skeletal muscles to contract and relax normally, sufficient levels of these minerals are needed. Apple cider vinegar enhances the absorption of calcium and magnesium from food, making them more available to take part in normal muscle contractions. Additionally, acetic acid in vinegar is broken down into acetate in the body. Acetate was found to increase calcium absorption in human distal colons and rectums in healthy human subjects.[93] In a rat model, acetic acid not only enhanced calcium absorption but also increased its retention.[94] A study in male rats found that when acetic acids levels were increased in the waste products in the cecum

NUTRITION

HEALTH

BEAUTY

HOME

of the large intestine, calcium and magnesium absorption and retention were significantly elevated.[95] Apple cider vinegar also increases iron absorption.[96] This is needed in the body to deliver oxygen to cells and is used to enhance energy and prevent muscle cramps from iron deficiency–induced muscle fatigue.

62. NoSEBLEEDS

Nosebleeds can start suddenly, and it can be quite alarming to watch blood pour out of the nasal passages of a child or elderly adult. Rest assured that most nosebleeds are relatively minor and not dangerous. When the tiny blood vessels near the surface of the skin in the nose become irritated due to dry air, nose picking, or trauma, they bleed into the nasal cavity and drip out of the nose. The majority of bleeds stop on their own, but to assist the process, sit upright and lean the head forward. Pinch the nostrils between two fingers for ten minutes. The blood should clot and the bleeding stop.

Keep apple cider vinegar on hand for the next time a nosebleed happens to a family member. Tear off a raspberry-size piece of a cotton ball and soak it in apple cider vinegar. Squeeze gently to remove any excess so it doesn't drip. Insert the cotton into the nostril that is bleeding, taking care not to put it in too far. Most bleeds happen from blood vessels near the front of the nasal passageways. Astringent properties of the gallic acid in vinegar will constrict the irritated tissue and stop the bleeding.

63. NUTRIENT ABSORPTION

Food provides the nutrients necessary to the body for growth, maintenance, and survival. Eating a diet rich in vitamins and minerals, complex carbohydrates, and good fats should provide the basic ingredients for a healthy, thriving individual. Sometimes, however, all this good food cannot be used to its full potential because the body is not able to completely digest and absorb the nutrients. One of the major reasons for poor nutrient absorption and nutrient deficiency is low stomach acid. This condition is extremely common, especially in older adults. Hydrochloric acid in the stomach is needed to begin breaking down protein in food. If levels of this acid are low, proteins are not properly digested and vitamin B12 and several minerals cannot be released from the protein. The partially digested protein molecules enter the intestines and either pass into the waste for secretion or into the blood where they are attacked as foreign particles. This leads to food allergies, food sensitivities, increased risk of infections, and colon toxicity.

To remedy the situation, consume a small glass of water with 1 teaspoon of apple cider vinegar fifteen minutes before a meal. This will increase the amount of acid in the stomach to aid in the breakdown of protein before it gets passed into the intestine, where nutrient absorption takes place. More apple cider vinegar may be needed if stomach acids are suspected to be very low or nonexistent. The vinegar can also increase the absorption of important minerals like calcium, magnesium, phosphorus, and iron. A study in male rats found that when acetic acid levels (the main acid in apple cider vinegar) were increased in the waste products in the cecum of the large intestine, calcium, magnesium, and phosphorus absorption and retention were significantly elevated.[97] Another study showed that acetic acid and malic acid found in apple cider vinegar both enhance iron absorption in a human cell line.[98] The importance of consuming nutrient-dense food and maintaining the body in a condition in which it can break down and absorb nutrients cannot be understated for a healthy and happy life.

64. PLANTAR FASCIITIS

This is the most common cause of heel pain. It is named after the plantar fascia, the thick band of tissue that runs along the bottom of the foot, from the heel to the toes. This tissue normally supports the arch of the foot, but repeated strain can cause tiny tears that lead to pain and swelling. Pain is most pronounced upon taking the first few steps in the morning or after standing or walking for long periods of time. Most cases can be resolved with rest, physical therapy, night splints, orthotics, and over-the-counter pain relievers. In more severe cases, steroid shots, shock wave therapy, or surgery are used.

Acetic acid, the main acid in apple cider vinegar, has been shown to be effective in the treatment of plantar fasciitis. In a double-blind, randomized, placebo-controlled trial, thirty-one patients were given either acetic acid, a corticosteroid hormone, or saline to treat the symptoms of their plantar fasciitis. Each treatment was combined with taping and administered through iontophoresis—the process of using low-volt electrical current to send the acid, hormone, or saline through the outermost layer of skin. The acetic acid treatment gave the best results with the greatest relief from stiffness and was equally as effective as the corticosteroid hormone at relieving pain.[99] For an at-home treatment, soak the foot in a warm bath of apple cider vinegar for fifteen minutes. Repeat each day until the condition improves.

65. POISON IVY ALLERGIC REACTION

A lucky 15 percent of the population is not allergic to poison ivy. That means 85 percent need to be extra cautious when outdoors in areas known to have the plant. Brushing up against the leaves, stems, or roots of the plant can transfer an oily resin called urushiol to the skin. Even if direct contact with the plant isn't made, touching pets, gardening tools, clothing, or other items that came into contact with the plant can transfer the urushiol. The resin quickly penetrates the skin, and symptoms develop within twelve to seventy-two hours. Redness, itching, swelling, and blisters that may weep and crust over are commonly found on the skin and last anywhere from one to three weeks. The rash is not contagious, but urushiol can be transferred from person to person. Washing the affected skin with mild soap and warm water to remove the resin will lessen the severity of the infection—or even prevent it if the resin is washed away before it has a chance to penetrate the skin. A poison ivy reaction is self-limiting and often goes away on its own, but if it is severe or an infection starts, corticosteroids and antibiotics are prescribed by a doctor.

As early as the 18th century, US medical practitioners used vinegar to treat cases of poison ivy.[100] This treatment has endured through the centuries and is still used as a natural household remedy today. Apple cider vinegar helps reduce the inflammation and itch caused by the poison ivy allergic rash. When the urushiol penetrates the skin, the immune system launches an attack against it and releases histamine and pro-inflammatory cytokines into the affected area of the skin. This causes the rash to develop and the skin to become swollen, red, and itchy. By preventing the release of these compounds, the reaction may not be as severe. Reducing swelling will lessen the pressure on the nerves and stop the itching sensation. Apple cider vinegar applied directly to the rash can be used to prevent a bacterial infection from making the condition worse. The acetic acid and the different phenolic acids in the vinegar are all antibiotics and have the ability to cross the bacterial cell membranes and destroy any bacteria that try to invade the skin at the rash site. Apply apple cider vinegar to a cotton ball and wash over the area, taking care to avoid any open blisters. This should help relieve the symptoms of poison ivy and may shorten the duration of the reaction.

66. SLOW METABOLISM

Chemical reactions in the body convert everything consumed into nutrients used to maintain good health and proper functioning of cells in the entire body. Some of these reactions break down compounds to be used as energy. Other reactions build compounds that the cells use to carry out their jobs and to grow and repair tissues. The vitamins and minerals in food play a crucial role in boosting metabolism. They act as enzymes to speed up reactions in the body that are necessary to produce energy for the body's functions. Without these enzymes, the reactions would be slow or stop altogether, causing a sluggish metabolism, which impacts health.

There are many reasons for a slow metabolism. With age, muscle mass declines and fat accounts for more body weight. Muscle burns more energy than fat. Women generally have higher percentages of fat in their bodies than men, so metabolism tends to be slower in women. People on diets may restrict their calories too much, causing their metabolism to slow down to conserve energy. Some conditions like an underactive thyroid or diabetes are associated with slow metabolisms, while certain medications and genetics play a role as well.

When the body does not have all the nutrients it needs to perform its metabolic functions to keep the body working properly, metabolism slows down because the vitamins, minerals, amino acids, or other substances are not available to drive the reactions. When this happens as a result of poor digestion due to low stomach acid, apple cider vinegar can help remedy the situation. When the stomach acid level is too low, proteins are not properly broken down. Amino acids, minerals, and vitamins that are bound in the proteins cannot be released for use in the body's metabolic processes. Drinking apple cider vinegar fifteen minutes before a meal can increase the level of acid in the stomach and aid in the process of protein digestion, releasing nutrients to be used in the body. Metabolism can move forward, and reactions can speed up. Metabolism is further improved by the acetic acid in the vinegar. It joins to an important coenzyme, CoA, that is central in the metabolism of carbohydrates and fats and produces energy for biochemical processes. Start with 1 teaspoon in a small glass of water. Gradually increase the amount of vinegar up to 2 tablespoons before each meal if stomach acid is very low.

67. SORE THROAT

A sore throat is pain, irritation, and itchiness of the throat that worsens upon swallowing. The glands of the neck might be swollen, the voice may be hoarse, and small white patches can even appear on the tonsils. The main culprits are viral and bacterial infections, but smoke, dry air, and allergies can cause a sore throat too. When the tissues lining the throat become irritated or infected, blood rushes to the area and brings with it germ-fighting cells. The blood vessels in the tissues swell, putting pressure on the nerve endings and causing pain. Sore throats from viral infections usually last five to seven days and are treated with over-the-counter pain relievers. Bacterial infections, like strep throat, require antibiotics.

Apple cider vinegar can be used to treat the symptoms and the cause of a sore throat. It can lower levels of histamines and pro-inflammatory cytokines in the body that cause inflammation and subsequent pain in blood vessels. This will make swallowing much less painful. Apple cider vinegar is also a strong topical remedy to rid the body of infections and can effectively attack both bacterial and viral sources. Taking apple cider vinegar will decrease the duration of infection; its antibacterial and antiviral acids attack the pathogens by crossing their cell walls, disrupting metabolic function and causing cell death. If the infection is severe and antibiotics are required, apple cider vinegar can still be used as a complement to bring extra fighting power. Mix a solution of half apple cider vinegar and half water and gargle once an hour for relief of symptoms.

. . . .

68. SUPPORTED IMMUNE SYSTEM

The immune system is the body's defense against bacteria, viruses, fungi, parasites, toxins, and allergens that could potentially invade the body and cause a lot of harm. It has a network of cells, tissues, and organs throughout the body that work around the clock and communicate when a threat is detected so it can mount a defense. Because the immune system is so busy, any help it can get is needed to prevent it from becoming overburdened. If this happens, disease can take over.

This is where apple cider vinegar steps in. It has antifungal, antiviral, and antibacterial properties,[101, 102] which can attack any of these invading organisms and spare the immune system from getting involved. The acetic acid and phenolic acids in apple cider vinegar are able to cross the pathogen's cell membranes, disrupt metabolic functions, and cause cell death. The acids are also antioxidants that can stop free radicals. These are responsible for damage to cells and tissues. They are unstable molecules actively looking for an electron. Free radicals attack the nearest stable molecule and steal one of their electrons, making that molecule a free radical. This begins a chain reaction of creating free radicals that ultimately can destroy the cell. The acids in apple cider vinegar

NUTRITION

HEALTH

BEAUTY

HOME

stabilize the free radicals by giving them one of their electrons. Damage is prevented, so the immune system doesn't have to clean up the aftereffects.

Finally, taking apple cider vinegar can help the liver, which is part of the immune system, by normalizing blood sugar levels.[103] This job usually falls to the liver and is a constant balancing act. When blood sugar levels are too high, it's up to the liver to take in the excess sugar, which it stores or converts to fat. All the extra work can stress the liver and prevent it from working optimally. The entire immune system suffers. If the immune system doesn't seem to be healing wounds quickly or if multiple colds take hold over the season, it might need a little help. Take 2 tablespoons of apple cider vinegar in 1 cup of water each day.

69. TOOTHACHE

Pain in or around a tooth that is sharp or throbbing is a toothache. The pain may be constant or present only when pressure is applied to the tooth and is generally a result of the tooth's nerve root becoming irritated. Swelling around the tooth and headaches sometimes occur. Some causes are tooth decay, damaged fillings, infected gums, trauma to the tooth, or teeth grinding. Dental treatment is often necessary to fix a damaged tooth. Over-the-counter pain medications are used to temporarily dull pain and inflammation.

An alternative to these pain medications, like ibuprofen or acetaminophen, is apple cider vinegar. This can be used to experience pain relief without the side effects. It contains an anti-inflammatory substance called gallic acid and can provide relief by inhibiting histamines and pro-inflammatory prostaglandins that cause inflammation, which compresses the nerve of the tooth and causes pain. If tooth decay is the issue, the antibacterial properties of the acids in the vinegar are effective in killing the bacteria and will prevent further decay. Apply apple cider vinegar to a cotton ball and place on the affected tooth.

70. VAGINITIS

Vaginitis is an inflammation of the vagina, affecting up to one-third of women during their lives. When the normal balance of bacteria or yeast in the vagina is altered, overgrowth of unwanted pathogens can infect the tissue lining the vagina and cause itching, pain, and abnormal discharge. Other types of vaginal infections are from parasites transmitted sexually or change in hormone levels. Antibiotics, antifungal ointments, antiprotozoal drugs, or estrogen can be prescribed, depending on the source of vaginal infection.

The symptoms of bacterial vaginitis have been successfully managed or cured by women using apple cider vinegar.[104] The acids in the vinegar can destroy the source of infection if it is bacterial or fungal. Acetic acid and the phenolic acids can penetrate the cell walls of bacteria, disrupt metabolic functions, and cause cell death. Yeast infections causing vaginitis are often from *Candida*. A 4 percent solution of vinegar has a significant reduction on *Candida* yeast and dramatically reduces their numbers.[105] The vinegar has anti-inflammatory properties that can reduce swelling, redness, and pain. Fill a sitz bath with warm water and add 1 cup of apple cider vinegar. Sit and relax in the bath for twenty minutes, allowing the solution to wash in and around the vagina.

71. WEIGHT LOSS

When the body accumulates too much body fat, it increases the risk of health problems like diabetes, heart disease, and certain cancers. Losing weight can improve or prevent any weight-induced conditions. Fat accumulates on the body when more calories are eaten than burned. The body stores these excess calories as fat. Exercising and eating a healthy diet with appropriate calorie intake will help burn the stored fat and reduce body weight.

During the weight-loss process, people often report reaching plateaus where they no longer seem to be able to continue losing weight despite continued efforts with exercise and dieting. This is because metabolism slows down as weight is lost. Apple cider vinegar can counteract this decrease in metabolism by supplementing the amount of acid in the stomach. People with low amounts of hydrochloric acid are unable to properly digest protein. Partially digested protein binds amino acids, vitamins, and minerals essential to the metabolic processes and makes them unavailable for use by the body. Without these key nutrients, metabolism has to slow down since it doesn't have the compounds needed to work. Taking apple cider vinegar fifteen minutes before meals can increase the amount of acid in the stomach to aid in protein digestion, nutrient availability, and, ultimately, a faster metabolism. Increased metabolism burns more fuel, resulting in weight loss. More fuel can also be burned when enough oxygen reaches the cells. Iron is needed to carry oxygen in red blood cells to the tissues of the body. Malic acid and acetic acid found in apple cider vinegar both enhance iron absorption.[106] Many people are deficient in iron, so their stores are not sufficient for maximal oxygen delivery to the cells and subsequent fuel consumption for energy. Greater iron levels can deliver more oxygen to the cells to burn more calories and help weight loss.

Apple cider vinegar also decreases daily intake of calories by approximately 200 to 275 kilocalories after a high glycemic load meal such as a bagel and juice, which translates into a monthly weight loss of 1 to 1 1/2 pounds.[107] In obese Japanese men, ingesting vinegar each day significantly reduced body weight, body mass index, visceral fat area, and waist circumference compared to the placebo group of men who did not consume vinegar.[108]

NUTRITION

HEALTH

BEAUTY

HOME

CHAPTER 3

··

BOOST YOUR BEAUTY

··

BEAUTIFUL SKIN

72. ACNE

Having clear skin gives confidence to face fears, take risks, and reach for goals. Waking up on the morning of a big presentation in front of a hundred colleagues and seeing acne has erupted across the chin can really make a person feel self-conscious, anxious, or even depressed. Acne is a skin condition that results in pimples, blackheads, whiteheads, cysts, nodules, and papules. It often appears on the face, but it can also show up on the neck, chest, back, upper arms, shoulder, and buttocks. Acne is the most common skin problem in the United States. It happens when dead skin cells stick together with sebum (oil) inside the pore. They become trapped. Bacteria living on the skin can sometimes get stuck in the pores with the dead skin cells. This provides a perfect breeding ground for them, and they quickly multiply. The skin becomes inflamed. If the acne goes deeper into the skin, a nodule or cyst forms. Typically, acne appears in teenagers and young adults, but it can affect anyone, even babies. Scars and dark spots on the skin can result. Mild acne can be treated with over-the-counter products that contain benzoyl peroxide or salicylic acid. It takes four to eight weeks of using the product for acne to clear. For best resolution, a dermatologist should treat more severe cases. Prescription-grade topical treatments, whole body treatments like antibiotics, or office procedures involving lasers, lights, or chemicals may be used.

Apple cider vinegar has a few mechanisms to help keep the skin clear, smooth, and acne-free. It lowers levels of histamines and pro-inflammatory cytokines in the body that cause inflammation and subsequent pain from compressed nerves. This helps reduce swelling, redness, and pain associated with large, rounded blemishes. They become less noticeable and bothersome to the individual. The antibacterial properties of apple cider vinegar destroy bacteria trapped in the pores to shorten the duration of the acne and support the immune system in fighting these germs. When antibiotics are prescribed, apple cider vinegar may be supplemented alongside them to provide extra bacteria-fighting power. And the treatment is super simple! Using a cotton ball soaked in apple cider vinegar to swipe over the acne can reduce the appearance of large, red blemishes and help clear the infection more quickly.

73. AGE SPOTS

Spending a lot of time outdoors is a healthy way to grow up, but all those years of sun exposure without sunscreen protection can cause the appearance of flat brown, gray, or black areas of pigmentation on the skin called age spots. They typically appear on the areas of the skin most exposed to the sun, like the face, hands, arms, chest, and shoulders. Ultraviolet radiation from the sun speeds up the production of melanin, creating a darker pigmentation of the skin known as a tan. After many years of sun exposure, melanin pigments can become clumped together, forming oval or round spots. These spots are generally harmless. Some people opt to treat them for cosmetic reasons. Prescription-strength creams containing retinol or hydroquinone are effective at fading the age spots. Microdermabrasion, laser treatments, chemical peels, and light therapy are also used.

In order to fade age spots, the treatment must penetrate the outermost layers of skin to reach the cells producing the melanin pigment. Applying apple cider vinegar topically to the skin allows the acids—in particular the acetic acid—to be absorbed and reach these cells. It is thought the acetic acid breaks apart the clumps of melanin, fading age spots over time. There are several ways in which apple cider vinegar is used to fade age spots. Some mix it with equal parts onion juice, with orange juice in a one to four ratio, or even by adding a few drops of the vinegar to a tablespoon of honey. All methods are applied directly to the age spots on the skin. Treatment can take from six weeks to six months, depending on the responsiveness of the individual. If any skin irritation occurs, try diluting the treatment further with water.

74. AGING

The process of getting older involves many changes in the body. Arteries stiffen, bones lose density, memory declines, skin thins, and wrinkles appear. The rate at which these processes take place varies from person to person. Genetics and illness play a role in when and how we age, but our diet and lifestyle significantly impact the process. There are many theories about aging, but the free radical theory is growing in popularity as an explanation. It is thought that free radicals are responsible for age-related damage of

cells and tissues. Free radicals are unstable molecules actively looking for an electron. They attack the nearest stable molecule and steal
one of their electrons, making that molecule a free radical as well.
This begins a chain reaction of creating free radicals that ultimately
can destroy the cell.

The key to stopping these free radicals lies in the presence of
antioxidants. The acids in apple cider vinegar are antioxidant compounds. These compounds sidle up to free radicals and give them
an electron. Now they are happy and leave neighboring molecules
alone. Cells and tissue continue to live, and the aging process is
slowed. This happens throughout the body, from the liver to the skin.
Consuming apple cider vinegar with water or applying it topically
will slow aging and give a healthier and more youthful appearance.

75. BRUISES

Often, bruises happen from events that go unnoticed, such as
bumping into a bedpost or catching a hip on the kitchen counter.
Others happen from vigorous exercise, bleeding disorders, or blood-
thinning medications. Elderly persons are more susceptible to
bruises because they have thinner skin that gives less support to the
blood vessels underneath. When the skin is injured, the blood cells
under the skin are damaged. They leak blood, which pools underneath the surface of the skin, giving rise to a tender and sometimes
painful black or blue mark. The bruise begins to heal and turns yellow or green. It eventually fades as the blood is reabsorbed. Ice and
later heat can be applied to the bruise to reduce swelling and improve circulation to the area.

NUTRITION

HEALTH

BEAUTY

HOME

To speed the healing of bruises, apply apple cider vinegar to a small cloth or cotton ball and place on the bruise for an hour. The swelling should reduce, along with any tenderness and pain. Gallic acid in apple cider vinegar is an anti-inflammatory and can inhibit the release of histamine and pro-inflammatory cytokines into the bruised area. These compounds produce swelling of the tissue. This compresses the pain-sensing nerves in the bruised area, and they fire, causing pain and tenderness. Apple cider vinegar is also an astringent. Applying it directly to the skin after trauma may help constrict tissues in the area and reduce bleeding. The result would be a smaller bruise with less healing time.

76. DEODORANT

Sweating is a natural function of the body, used to reduce body heat. Sweat itself is odorless. The warm, moist environment, however, is a breeding ground for bacteria, and they thrive in the armpit in these conditions. The bacteria break down keratin proteins on the surface of the skin and produce odor-causing fatty acids and ammonia. To reduce armpit odor, wash regularly and keep the armpit dry. Most people use antiperspirants to reduce sweating or deodorants to mask odor.

Because sweating is a natural process to regulate body temperature and remove toxins from the body, allowing the body to sweat is recommended. Deodorants can help mask odor for a period of time, but bacteria can overpower even the most pungent scents. The best way to be odor-free is to make sure the bacteria don't have a chance to grow in the armpits. Apple cider vinegar should keep away any offending odors. Soak a cotton ball in apple cider vinegar and swipe over the armpit area. Acetic acid and the phenolic acids in the vinegar are antibacterial. They cross the bacterial cell membranes, disrupt metabolic functions, and cause cell death. This prevents them from producing odor-causing compounds. As the day wears on, reapply as needed.

77. DIAPER RASH

When the skin under a diaper gets chafed or irritated, it may become red and tender. This commonly occurs in babies between nine and twelve months old when their diets change and their bowel movements become more acidic. It can also be caused by bacterial or fungal infections. Changing diapers often to prevent wetness or acidic wastes from irritating the skin or using non-allergenic detergents, soaps, lotions, and wipes can help prevent or lessen the incidence of diaper rash. If a rash persists despite these precautions, a doctor may prescribe hydrocortisone cream, antibiotics, or antifungal lotion. The rash should go away in a few days.

If the rash is caused by a bacterial or fungal infection, apple cider vinegar can help. Both acetic acid and the phenolic acids are antibacterial and antifungal and are effective at destroying the pathogens. The acids can cross the cell membranes of bacteria and disrupt metabolic functions, causing cell death. Significant fungicidal activity against *Candida*—the common fungus responsible for some diaper rash infections—was found in a laboratory study using a 4 percent solution of apple cider vinegar.[109] The vinegar also has anti-inflammatory properties that can reduce swelling,

NUTRITION

HEALTH

BEAUTY

HOME

redness, and pain. The rash should clear up quickly, and the baby should be more comfortable. Dip a washcloth in a solution of half apple cider vinegar and half water. Gently swipe over the rash. Avoid any broken skin. Repeat each time the diaper is changed.

78. ECZEMA

This is a group of medical conditions that cause the skin to become itchy and inflamed. It is often accompanied by asthma or hay fever and is common in infants, affecting up to 20 percent, although most children outgrow eczema by their tenth birthday. It also affects about 3 percent of adults and children who experience it on and off throughout their lives. During a flare-up, the skin is itchy, thickened, dry, and scaly. The skin may be red or brown, and pigmentation could be affected. There are many triggers that cause flare-ups, like scratching, hot showers, stress, clothing, or allergens. Nearly all people with eczema have *Staphylococcus aureus* bacteria on the skin, which multiply rapidly if they find their way into the skin. If this happens, symptoms worsen. Creams and oral drugs to control itching and inflammation can help manage symptoms, and antibiotics can help clear up an infection.

The main goal for treatment of eczema is to relieve itching, since scratching can lead to infection. Apple cider vinegar applied topically can do this. Gallic acid in the vinegar is an anti-inflammatory and can stop the release of histamine and pro-inflammatory cytokines. This means the tissue swelling will decrease and no longer press on the nerves that cause itching. If *Staphylococcus aureus* does manage to cause an infection, the acids in apple cider vinegar can cross their cell membranes, disrupt their functions, and cause cell death. The infection should clear. Wash the affected skin with a cloth dipped in apple cider vinegar. Avoid the eye area and any open wounds. Repeat as necessary to relieve itching and improve the infection.

79. EXFOLIATION

Exfoliating on a regular basis keeps the skin glowing and fresh and is a healthy habit to get into. The process removes dead skin cells from the outermost layer of the skin to expose the new, radiant skin underneath. This skin is smooth and soft and immediately makes a person look younger. Exfoliating is usually done by either mechanical means with a loofah, pumice stone, body brush, or exfoliating gloves or by chemical means at a spa or doctor's office. Most take care to exfoliate the face, but doing the entire body can make your skin feel alive and look luminous. Moreover, it allows moisturizer to penetrate deeper into the skin for better hydration.

Part of the exfoliating process is using a facial or body scrub. There are many available in stores, but an inexpensive and very effective way to remove dead skin and start the rejuvenation process is to make a scrub at home with apple cider vinegar. Try mixing 1 teaspoon of organic apple cider vinegar with an equal amount of raw local honey and 5 teaspoons of sugar. Apply to the skin and scrub gently. Rinse with warm water. The apple cider vinegar contains malic acid, an alpha hydroxy acid. These acids work by ungluing the cells from one another and causing them to slough off. This process gets rid of dead skin cells and thins the outermost layer of skin, allowing for fresh, new cells to come to the surface, stimulating the production of new cells underneath. Apple cider vinegar has antibacterial properties, so any skin condition, like acne, will benefit from destruction of bacterial cells to allow the skin to heal. It's important to protect the new cells that the exfoliating process brings to the surface. Apple cider vinegar does just this. It contains antioxidants and can defend the skin against free radical–inflicted sun damage.

80. FOOT ODOR

Smelly feet can be embarrassing, but they are preventable with a little care. The feet have more sweat glands than anywhere else on the body. They typically release about a pint of sweat a day, most of which evaporates. If the moisture is trapped, however, bacteria on the skin of the foot feed on the sweat. The combination causes the bad odor that is associated with smelly feet. To prevent this from happening, wash the feet every day and dry thoroughly. Wear cotton socks and leather or canvas shoes, which are more breathable than other fabrics. Antiperspirants or deodorants can also be used to prevent the foot from sweating or masking odor. The same ones used under the arms can be used on the foot.

Sweating releases toxins from the body and helps regulate body temperature, so the use of antiperspirants on the foot should only be employed if all else fails. Instead, try washing the foot with a cloth dipped in apple cider vinegar. The acids in the vinegar have antibacterial properties that will reduce bacterial cell numbers on the foot so that they cannot convert sweat into odor-causing agents. The smell of the vinegar will quickly fade and not be carried on the foot. Try to keep feet dry and reapply vinegar as needed for extra odor protection.

81. HAND SANITIZER

Hand sanitizers are alcohol-based cleansing products that are touted as an effective way to wash hands in the absence of soap and water. Simply rub a small amount over the hands and let dry. The oil on the surface of the hands is stripped away and presumably with it any bacteria. Most companies claim their products kill 99.9 percent of germs, although these numbers are obtained from studies on inert surfaces, not on hands. The Centers for Disease Control and Prevention recommend washing hands with soap and water as the best way to remove microbes in most situations, but alcohol-based hand sanitizers can be used as an alternative when necessary.

When washing with soap and water is not possible, rubbing apple cider vinegar over the hands can be used as an alternative to get rid of germs. It has antibacterial, antiviral, and antifungal properties that can attack any pathogen on the hands, leading to a reduction in their numbers. It is known that vinegar destroys bacteria, viruses, and mold on the surface of food so they can't multiply. It is plausible that they can perform in a similar way on the hands. The acidity of the vinegar is thought to break down the microorganism's proteins, thereby destroying them. It works so well that solutions containing 10 percent vinegar are able to reduce bacteria on strawberries by 90 percent and significantly reduce the number of viruses after a two-minute wash.[110] Applying vinegar to rocket leaves and spring onions significantly reduced *Salmonella* cells on the vegetables. Combining the vinegar with lemon juice brought the bacteria count down to undetectable levels.[111] Apple cider vinegar can be used as a substitute for commercial alcohol-based hand sanitizers. It will eliminate germs and moisturize the skin rather than dry it out by stripping its oils.

82. MOISTURIZER

Keeping skin hydrated and moisturized plumps it up and gives the appearance of youth. Adding a facial moisturizer to a daily beauty routine is highly recommended, even for those with oily skin. Oily skin still needs moisture; otherwise, it will begin to look sallow and tired. There are different moisturizers available for different skin types. Oily skin is prone to acne and breakouts and does well with a light moisturizer to protect it from harsh cleansing products. Dry skin needs a heavier oil-based moisturizer to restore hydration. Normal skin benefits from lotions containing lightweight oils, and sensitive skin should use products without allergens and with soothing ingredients in them.

A few drops of apple cider vinegar can be combined with an equal amount of jojoba oil and used to moisturize the face. This can be used for all skin types because it won't clog pores, is lightweight, and is very moisturizing. Malic acid in the vinegar is an alpha hydroxy acid and is able to attract moisture and penetrate the skin. This brings the moisture deep within, plumping up the skin and making it look younger and more supple. It reduces the appearance of fine lines and wrinkles. Malic acid is also a good exfoliator. It removes dead skin cells and stimulates the production of new cells underneath. By providing moisture to these new cells and allowing them to rise to the surface of the skin, the overall tone, smoothness, and elasticity of the skin appears fresh and healthy.

83. SKIN TONER

There are different kinds of toner for different skin types. Some are moisturizing and soothe the skin by adding hydration, oils, and extracts. Others cleanse and refresh the skin by removing oils, tightening the skin, and shrinking the appearance of pores. Choose a toner that benefits the condition of your facial skin.

Fortunately, apple cider vinegar works well with all skin types. If the skin tends to be oily, apple cider vinegar can prevent shine by removing oils and make the skin appear younger and fresher. The gallic acid in the vinegar is an astringent and shrinks skin tissue, so pores and fine lines appear less visible. If the skin tends to be dry, malic acid—an alpha hydroxy acid in apple cider vinegar— gently removes dead skin cells and stimulates the production of new cell growth. In addition, its antioxidants prevent free radicals generated from toxins and the sun's ultraviolet rays from damaging skin cells. The facial skin retains a brighter, more radiant appearance. After cleansing the skin, add a diluted amount of apple cider vinegar to a cotton ball. Swipe across the entire face, avoiding the delicate eye area. If the skin is sensitive, dilute the apple cider vinegar with more water. Follow with a moisturizer.

NUTRITION

HEALTH

BEAUTY

HOME

84. SUNBURN

Sitting outside in the sun for too long without protection from sunscreen can cause the skin to burn. The ultraviolet rays of the sun penetrate the skin and increase the rate of melanin production. This is the body's way of protecting the skin from the damaging effects of the sun, but when exposure is too long or the rays too intense, melanin is not enough, and the skin burns. It becomes red, painful, and swollen. It is hot to the touch and may form small, fluid-filled blisters. Tanning lamps can burn the skin in the same way the sun does. Even the sun's rays that reflect off the surface of water, sand, ice, and snow can give a sunburn. Cloudy days emit 80 percent of the sun's ultraviolet rays, so caution is needed for outdoor activities on these days as well. Sunburned skin begins to heal itself within a few days. Pain relievers and corticosteroids are often used for pain and to control itching.

While nothing but time can be used to remove the sunburn, the symptoms can be managed with apple cider vinegar. Take a bath with 1 cup of apple cider vinegar added to soothe the skin and stop itching. Gallic acid in apple cider vinegar is an anti-inflammatory and reduces the swelling of the burned skin tissue. This relieves pressure on the nerves responsible for the itching sensation, so they no longer fire and the itch is relieved. When swelling is reduced, pain and tenderness decrease. Sloughing off the damaged skin will also reduce itching. Malic acid in apple cider vinegar is an excellent exfoliant and can help remove dead skin cells and stimulate the growth of new cells. Taking baths with apple cider vinegar can speed healing time and increase comfort by reducing itching and pain.

85. WARTS

Warts are small skin growths caused by the human papillomavirus (HPV). They are usually flesh-colored and contain small black dots, which are actually clotted blood vessels. The hands and the fingers are the most common areas where they are found, which is not surprising since the virus is contagious. If warts occur on the soles of the feet, they are called plantar warts. Most warts go away on their own, but it may take a year or two. Many people find them embarrassing and opt to get rid of them using salicylic acid medications, freezing, or laser treatments. These can cause pain, blistering, and scarring.

Apple cider vinegar can be used to effectively remove common and plantar warts. The phenolic acids and acetic acid in the vinegar have antiviral properties and are able to destroy HPV after several applications. Tear off a small piece of a cotton ball, just enough to cover the wart but not the surrounding skin. Soak it in apple cider vinegar and squeeze out any excess. Lightly apply a thin layer of petroleum jelly on the normal skin around the wart to protect it from the acid in the vinegar. Secure the cotton over the wart and keep in place with a bandage. Do this at night, and sleep with the bandage on. Remove in the morning. Repeat each night until the wart disappears. This may take anywhere from several days to several weeks.

NUTRITION

HEALTH

BEAUTY

HOME

NUTRITION

HEALTH

BEAUTY

HOME

GORGEOUS HAIR AND NAILS

86. CLEANSE AND CLARIFY

Sebum is the natural oil produced by the skin that coats the hair follicle and gives it shine. Too much sebum can make the hairs stick together and cause the hair to look greasy and dull. Sebum repels water; washing with only water will not remove the excess sebum built up on the hair. Shampoos or other substances that can remove the sebum from the hair follicle are necessary to cleanse the hair. Many shampoos strip the oils from the hair, however, without adding back moisture. This causes the hair to become dry, brittle, and frizzy.

Using apple cider vinegar to cleanse the hair will allow the excess sebum to be removed as well as any product buildup that weighs the hair down and makes it look limp and lifeless. The vinegar locks moisture in the strands and seals the cuticles, allowing for smooth, soft, and shiny hair. It is able to do this because the vinegar is acidic and can counter the effects of alkaline products used on the hair. It brings the pH back down to its naturally mild acidic state. A spray bottle filled with 1/2 cup of apple cider vinegar and 4 cups of water can be kept in the shower and used in place of shampoo to cleanse and clarify the hair. Spray liberally on the hair and gently massage thoroughly into the scalp and hair. Be sure to avoid the eyes. Rinse after a few minutes. This same treatment is an excellent conditioner to add manageability and shine to the hair.

87. CONDITION AND SHINE

There are about one hundred thousand to one hundred and fifty thousand hairs on the human head. Those are a lot of strands to take care of! Each strand of hair consists of three layers, with the outer layer, or cuticle, protecting the inner two layers. When the hair is healthy, the scales of the cuticle overlap tightly and protect the inner layers. When it becomes damaged, however, the scales of the cuticle loosen and separate, exposing the layers underneath. The hair looks dry and dull and may break easily. Now the inner layers can become damaged from exposure to the UV rays of the sun, heat, pollution, chlorine, or any of the array of chemicals found in hair products and treatments.

To add shine and lock in moisture, rinse apple cider vinegar through the hair after washing. A spray bottle with 1/2 cup of vinegar and 4 cups of water can be kept in the shower and used twice a week. Massage the solution through the hair and rinse after a few minutes. The vinegar closes the hair cuticle, locking in moisture. The closed cuticle is smoother, softer, and has the ability to reflect light, making it shine. A closed cuticle also prevents split ends, so the hair is more flexible, has more body, and looks healthier.

NUTRITION

HEALTH

BEAUTY

HOME

88. DANDRUFF

Dandruff is a chronic condition marked by the flaking of skin cells on the scalp. They are visible as white, oily-looking flakes of skin on the hair and shoulders. It is not a dangerous condition, but it can be embarrassing for some people. Dandruff is usually worse in the fall and winter when the scalp is subjected to the drier, cooler outdoor air and heated indoor air, which depletes moisture in the skin. It can be caused by not shampooing enough, which results in dead skin cells mixing with oils. This causes a buildup and subsequent shedding of these cells as dandruff.

Yeast on the scalp can irritate some people and cause an overproduction of skin cells, which flake off as dandruff. Dry skin can cause smaller, drier flakes to appear. One of the most common causes of dandruff is seborrheic dermatitis. This is a condition in which oily skin is covered in flaky white or yellow scales. Mild cases are easy to treat with daily cleansing to reduce oil and skin cell buildup. Other cases are more difficult and may need medicated shampoos. Some shampoos contain antifungal and antibacterial agents to kill the microbes. Others work by slowing the death rate of skin cells to reduce buildup and flaking.

If the source of dandruff is yeast or the fungus causing seborrheic dermatitis, then massaging a diluted solution of apple cider vinegar into the scalp for ten minutes will help reduce the overproduction of skin cells. Apple cider vinegar has acids that destroy yeast and fungal cells. The amount of itching and dandruff produced will be greatly reduced or even entirely stopped. Its anti-inflammatory compound can reduce irritation of the scalp that causes red and tender skin, other symptoms associated with these infections. If dry skin is the culprit, apple cider vinegar can help here, too. It can exfoliate the skin, removing dead skin cells that are often the source of itchy skin. Exfoliation encourages new, healthy cells to be produced. The vinegar treatment is a one-step process that can be used to treat dandruff, to cleanse, and to condition the hair. Use at least three times a week to maintain results.

89. NAiL FUNGUS

Fungal infections are extremely common and can infect any part of the body. When fungus targets the fingernails or toenails, white or yellow spots may begin to appear. These spots then merge to form patches and spread out. The nails become thicker, brittle, or discolored, and the edges start to crumble. The symptoms occur slowly and may eventually result in the nail detaching from the skin and falling off.

Fungal infections can actually be a sign of *Candida* overgrowth in the body. *Candida albicans* is a very common fungus in humans and can grow out of control in people with weakened or compromised immune systems. The good bacteria in the gut cannot compete with *Candida* and a systemic invasion may begin, which can show up as a fungal infection of the nails. Over-the-counter treatments are available, but they are not always effective and the chance of reoccurrence is high. Prescribed oral antifungal drugs can be used that allow new growth of the nail to be fungus-free. This is a slow process and may cause a variety of side effects from a skin rash to liver disease. Medicated polishes and creams are used, but these can take a year to get rid of the fungus. The nail can also be surgically removed, but it grows back slowly.

Apple cider vinegar is an antifungal agent and can be used topically in the treatment of fungal infections. Fungal infections cause the pH of the nail and surrounding skin to become more alkaline. This works to the advantage of the fungus, because it thrives under such conditions. Apple cider vinegar is acidic and can lower the pH of the nail and skin enough to kill the fungus but not enough to damage the skin. Soak the toes in a footbath of half vinegar and half water. Do this at least once a day for thirty minutes. Completely dry the foot after. Continue to do this daily until the nail grows out and is replaced by a healthy fungus-free nail.

TERRIFIC TEETH

90. CLEAN DENTURES

Gum disease, tooth decay, and injury can all damage teeth to the point where they fall out or need to be removed. Dentures can replace missing teeth, improve facial appearance, and recover the ability to eat and speak. Complete dentures replace all the teeth in the mouth, while partial dentures replace only the teeth that are missing. Dentures should be removed at night and cleaned with a soft bristle toothbrush to remove food, plaque, bacteria, and yeast.

They should be stored in water overnight to prevent the dentures from drying out and warping. If dentures are not cleaned properly, they can cause irritation of the gums and bad breath.

Brushing dentures does remove food and plaque, but it is not very effective in removing bacteria and yeasts. If a disinfecting agent is not used in addition to brushing, the denture wearer runs the risk of infection of the mucosal membranes in the mouth. Both undiluted vinegar and vinegar diluted by 50 percent significantly reduced the number of bacteria on dentures compared to tap water alone.[112] Even a small amount of vinegar in water was found to be effective.

Candida is commonly found in the mouth. If left alone, it multiplies and thrives on the gums underneath the dentures. This causes a condition known as denture-induced stomatitis, which is an inflammation and redness of the gums. Soaking overnight in a 10 percent vinegar solution reduces *Candida* numbers on dentures.[113] The acetic acid and phenolic acids found in apple cider vinegar are antibacterial and antifungal and are responsible for the elimination of the pathogens.

91. MOUTHWASH

Using mouthwash as part of an oral hygiene regimen is optional, but many choose to include it. Most mouthwashes are antiseptic and are used to decrease the microbes in the mouth to prevent cavities, gingivitis, and bad breath. Others are advertised as reducing inflammation, pain, or dry mouth caused by infection or disease. About 20 milliliters of mouthwash is gargled for thirty seconds or more then spit out.

If bad breath is a problem, using apple cider vinegar as a mouthwash can remove the bacteria from the mouth and stop their metabolic byproducts from emitting offensive odors. It can also be used to eliminate much of the *Candida* yeast in the mouth to prevent localized and systemic infections that can spread to other areas of the body. For those using mouthwash to reduce inflammation of the gums, gallic acid in apple cider vinegar can prevent the release of specific compounds responsible for tissue swelling. Inflammation may be reduced and, along with it, pain. Tissue swelling compresses the pain-sensing nerves, causing them to fire. Release of this pressure would calm the nerve. The vinegar should be diluted with water and gargled before brushing.

92. TEETH WHITENER

Bright, white teeth make for a beautiful smile and give a younger and healthier appearance. There are many products in stores that claim to whiten teeth. Whitening toothpastes remove surface stains with mild abrasive agents and can achieve about one shade of difference. Whitening gels, strips, and trays contain hydrogen peroxide or other bleaching agents, which lighten deep within the tooth. Results usually last about four months. Some mouthwashes contain ingredients to whiten teeth, but they are less effective and results are often not seen for twelve weeks. Dentists can also dramatically whiten teeth in their offices in one visit. Tooth sensitivity and tissue irritation are a few side effects of the bleaching process.

Dilute a tablespoon of apple cider vinegar in a cup of water and swish around the mouth for one to two minutes. Rinse with water to remove the acid and the vinegar flavor from the mouth. The acid in the vinegar lifts stains from the teeth without harming the enamel. Like commercial whitening mouthwashes, this treatment works slowly over time, but consistent use will result in a brighter smile. According to *Reader's Digest*, up to 78 percent of people experience tooth sensitivity when whitening with products that use forms of peroxide.[114] Apple cider vinegar can be a gentle alternative to whiten teeth without sensitivity, allowing for daily use and no pain.

NUTRITION

HEALTH

BEAUTY

HOME

CHAPTER 4

BOOST YOUR HOME

93. DESCALE COFFEEMAKER

Hardworking coffeemakers brew cup after cup of java each morning and, sometimes, throughout the day. The water used by the majority of households is hard, though, and contains high amounts of minerals, especially calcium and magnesium. When the coffeemaker heats this water, the minerals precipitate out of the water and form a crust or scale inside the machine. While hard water is generally harmless to our health, it can change the flavor of freshly brewed coffee. Many people immensely enjoy the flavor of coffee, so an unpleasant taste can be very disappointing. Depending on how hard the water is, cleaning the coffeemaker each month or every other month can remove the scale and bring back the true flavor of that morning cup of joe.

Running a solution of half apple cider vinegar and half water through the machine will dissolve the scale so it can be washed out of the machine and no longer affect the flavor of the coffee. It is the acid in the vinegar that is responsible for this action, so a low-cost vinegar that doesn't contain the Mother is perfectly acceptable to use in this situation. After adding the solution to the water reservoir, run two brew cycles, then let the solution sit in the coffeemaker for an hour. Continue to run cycles after that time to remove the vinegar. Repeat until no vinegar smell remains. What is left is a clean, well-functioning machine to brew a perfect cup of coffee.

94. ELIMINATE CAT URINE ODOR

Cats can be very possessive and will urinate on carpets, furniture, drapes, clothes, and walls if they feel jealous, upset, or insecure. These odors are very difficult to remove and give off a strong, offensive odor. Cat urine is made up of mostly water, but other chemicals, principally ammonia, impart the overwhelming smell. Cats are often prone to bladder infections, and bacteria in the urine also get excreted and contaminate the area. A study published by the *Journal of the American Veterinary Association* found *Escherichia coli* (some species cause diarrhea, anemia, kidney failure, or urinary tract infection), Staphylococcus (may cause mild skin irritations or, if severe, sepsis), *Streptococcus* (some species cause meningitis, respiratory infections, and urinary tract infections), *Cornebacterium* (some species cause diphtheria), and *Flavobacterium* (some species cause meningitis in infants) in the urine of clinically normal cats.[115] These can be transferred to humans on contact and pose a health risk.

It is best to try to remove cat urine as soon as possible. Blot with paper towels to soak up any liquid. Spray a solution of half apple cider vinegar and half water directly on the stain, making sure to use enough to reach all layers, including the padding of carpets. After twenty minutes, blot the area again and let the vinegar dry completely. Vinegar is an acid and works to neutralize ammonia, which is a base. The reaction produces water and ammonium acetate—a salt. Breaking down ammonia eliminates odor and the visibility of

NUTRITION

HEALTH

BEAUTY

HOME

the stain. Vinegar also contains antibacterial acids that can destroy bacteria by interfering with their metabolism, causing cell death. This can prevent the spread of a bacterial infection to members of the family.

95. FABRIC SOFTENER

Adding fabric softener sheets to the dryer or liquids in the washing machine can reduce the static charge of clothing and soften clothes. Unfortunately, fabric softener can build up on clothes over time and reduce the flame resistance, particularly with fleece and flannel. Caution should be used when washing those items. Also, many fabric softeners contain chemicals that are toxic to humans and the environment. They coat the clothing with a layer of these chemicals. They can cause asthma, disrupt hormone function, and induce allergic reactions in sensitive individuals. The University of Washington did a study on contaminants found in the air from laundry products and discovered that they contained up to twenty chemicals, including ones that were thought to be carcinogens.[116]

Natural products that don't harm our health and preserve the environment are both personally kind and socially responsible. Adding 1/2 cup of apple cider vinegar to a load of laundry during the rinse cycle or in the machine's fabric softener dispenser can be used as a replacement for commercial liquid softeners. The vinegar removes soap and residue on the clothes, which is what causes clothes to become stiff over time. Vinegar can also dissolve mineral buildup in the machine to keep it working optimally. There is no need to worry about clothes coming out smelling like vinegar. The scent is washed away and does not stick to the clothes. And if you find yourself missing the pleasing smell that traditional fabric softeners leave, add a few drops of essential oils with the vinegar.

96. FRUIT AND VEGETABLE WASH

Farming practices in the growing of fruits and vegetables for commercial consumption use many different chemicals at various stages of the growing process. They are added to the soil in which the produce is grown and can be taken up and stored in the produce as they grow. The seeds, leaves, stems, and roots are often coated with pesticides to prevent them from being eaten or becoming diseased. During processing, more chemicals are added to increase size or accelerate ripening. All these chemicals accumulate on and within the produce and enter the body when ingested. These can harm the nervous, liver, kidney, and respiratory systems or be implicated in diseases like cancer.

Eating organic food can lessen the chemical load in food; however, organic produce still contains chemicals.[117] Organic farmers have the option of using chemical sprays and powders on their crops, but they must be derived from natural sources. Some of these are just as dangerous as synthetic chemicals. It is advisable to wash all produce before eating it. Apple cider vinegar can be used to rinse away pesticide residue and destroy bacteria, viruses, or fungi adhering to the surface. Soak produce in a solution of 1 tablespoon apple cider vinegar in 1 cup of water. Let the vegetables or fruit sit for five minutes, then rinse thoroughly. Discard the water.

97. FRUIT FLY TRAP

Fruit flies tend to invade homes during the warmer months of the year and typically get carried in on fruits and vegetables brought home from the grocery store. It is common to be seemingly free of fruit flies one day and bombarded with them the next. They breed very quickly and lay about four hundred eggs in ripe or rotting fruit or vegetables left on the counter. If no produce is around, they will breed in empty bottles, trash cans, cleaning rags, and garbage disposals. The eggs can hatch into larvae in as little as twelve hours under ideal temperatures. They feed on microorganisms and fermented sugars. When they become adults, the cycle begins over. Fruit flies are mainly nuisance pests, but they do have the potential of spreading bacteria to surfaces that they touch, like food, countertops, glasses, and dishes.

Getting rid of fruit flies requires some detective work. Discard all overripe, unrefrigerated food. Cover drains and garbage disposals. Put all empty bottles, jars, and jugs into the recycling bin outside the house. Take composting outside as well. Catch adults using a fruit fly trap made with apple cider vinegar. A simple fruit fly trap is made by taking a small glass and adding a few tablespoons of vinegar. Cover the top of the glass tightly with plastic wrap. With a toothpick, poke about ten holes in the plastic wrap. Leave the glass undisturbed in the kitchen or another area where the fruit flies seem to be. The flies are attracted to fermented sugar and will flock to the glass. They slip in through the tiny holes in the plastic wrap and cannot find their way out. Doing this over a few days should capture all the adults.

98. KILL WEEDS

In nature, no plant is a weed. People try to control nature to produce commercial crops, vegetable gardens, and varied landscaping. Plants that encroach on these areas and affect the viability of domesticated plants are considered weeds. They are unwanted, and considerable time and expense is expended trying to eradicate them. Weeds are persistent and adaptable, so getting rid of them can be very challenging.

Those that love tending personal gardens may spend hours each week pulling up weeds. Others use chemicals to selectively kill weeds but leave the intended plants unharmed. This route puts dangerous chemicals in the soil and air and can be harmful to family members and pets. A time-efficient and green method to kill weeds is to use apple cider vinegar. Fill an old gallon jug three-quarters full with vinegar. Add to this 3/4 cup of salt and 1 ounce of liquid dish soap. Spray directly on the weeds, being careful not to spray surrounding plants or grass. This application is nonselective and will damage any plant it contacts. The acetic acid in the vinegar destroys the plants. The dish soap is a surfactant and allows the vinegar to stick to the surface of the plant longer so it can do its work. The salt enters the plant and draws away water. It can take a day or two for the vinegar solution to kill the weeds, and a second or third application may be necessary for very hardy species.

NUTRITION

HEALTH

BEAUTY

HOME

99. REMOVE FLEAS FROM PETS

Fleas are small, copper-colored pests that live in warm, humid environments and feed on blood. They have strong hind legs and can jump onto pets from anywhere they can be found, whether it's other animals or from the environment. Fleas don't like light, so look on pets' bellies, on their hind legs, or deep within their fur to detect the fleas. Small, pepper-like flakes are telltale signs of a flea infestation; these are the feces from the flea. Fleas live for several weeks on pets and lay hundreds of eggs. The eggs can fall off pets and land on carpets, on furniture, on drapes, or even in floor cracks. They develop into larvae and feed on organic matter. As adults, they hop onto the nearest host. The bite of the flea causes itching in pets, and if the animal is allergic to the saliva of the flea, then skin infections, inflammation, and hair loss can result. Prescription pills or medicated shampoos can rid pets of fleas. Some dishwashing liquid is commonly used as well.

Apple cider vinegar can be used to reduce itching and repel fleas. Bathe pets with liquid dish detergent and rinse with apple cider vinegar. The liquid detergent kills the fleas, and the apple cider vinegar prevents a re-infestation. Fleas do not like the scent or flavor of the vinegar and won't remain on the animal. Dab apple cider vinegar on the back of the pet's neck each day for continued protection. The gallic acid in the apple cider vinegar will also help reduce itching by attenuating the allergic response and preventing the itch-specific nerves from firing. As a bonus, the vinegar rinse will make the pet's coat soft and shiny.

100. RINSE AID FOR DISHES

Most families dirty enough dishes to run the dishwasher at least once, if not several times, each day. Commercial rinse aids are often used to remove water spots from glasses and dishes. However, they are not environmentally friendly. Many contain toxic ingredients that get washed down the drain and into waterways that feed into rivers, lakes, streams, and oceans. They can kill aquatic life or have health effects on humans such as skin irritations, allergies, or cancer. They can affect the nervous system, digestive system, urinary tract, eyes, or reproductive system.

For a green alternative to commercial detergents, put 1/2 cup of apple cider vinegar on the top rack of the dishwasher. As the dishes are being washed, the vinegar gets mixed in with the water during the rinse cycle. The vinegar eliminates hard-water spots on glasses and dishes, and they come out sparkling clean. Don't worry about the vinegar smell; it doesn't stick to the dishes, and all traces of the smell are washed away.

101. STREAK-FREE WINDOWS

Clean windows allow the sun to shine through and give the homeowner a clear view of the outside. Sometimes, windows appear clean until the sun hits them in just the right way and they appear streaked with a film. Every pass of the cloth is etched in the glass, giving the window a dirty look. This can be frustrating for

NUTRITION

HEALTH

BEAUTY

HOME

the homeowner, who wants crystal-clear windows and takes pains-taking efforts to achieve this. Many commercial brands of window cleaners promise to be streak-free, but that isn't always the case.

Fill a spray bottle with a solution of half apple cider vinegar and half water. Spray on the windows and wipe with a microfiber cloth to ensure no lint remains. If some spots are resistant, dip a cloth in undiluted vinegar and rub directly over the spot. The acids in the vinegar break down dirt and leftover detergents that accumulate on the glass surface. If streaks remain after the first wash, reapply. These streaks are not the fault of the vinegar but of residue left over from commercial products previously applied to the glass. The result should be clean, clear windows that sparkle in the sun.

NOTES

1. Johnston, Carol S., and Cindy A. Gaas. 2006. "Vinegar: medicinal uses and antiglycemic effect." *Medscape General Medicine* 8 (2): 61.
2. The Online Archive of American Folk Medicine. Available at http://ahrt.ucla.edu.
3. Dabija, Adriana, and Cristian Aurel Hatnean. 2014. "Study concerning the quality of apple vinegar obtained through classical method." *Journal of Agroalimentary Processes and Technologies* 20 (4): 304–10. http://www.journal-of-agroalimentary.ro/admin/articole/93100L47_Vol_20(4)_2014_304_310.pdf.
4. The Natural Medicines site. Available at https://naturalmedicines.therapeuticresearch.com.
5. The United States Department of Agriculture Agricultural Research Service Food Composition Databases. Available at https://ndb.nal.usda.gov/ndb/.
6. Hill, L. L., L. H. Woodruff, J. C. Foote, and M. Barreto-Alcoba. 2005. "Esophageal injury by apple cider vinegar tablets and subsequent evaluation of products." *Journal of the American Dietetic Association* 105: 1141–4.
7. The Natural Medicines site, https://naturalmedicines.therapeuticresearch.com.
8. The Natural Medicines site, https://naturalmedicines.therapeuticresearch.com.
9. Shishehbor, F., A. Mansoori, A. R. Sarkaki, M. T. Jalali, and S. M. Latifi. 2008. "Apple cider vinegar attenuates lipid profile in normal and diabetic rats." *Pakistan Journal of Biological Sciences* 11 (23): 2634–8.
10. Johnston, C. S., I. Steplewska, C. A. Long, L. N. Harris, and R. H. Ryals. 2010. "Examination of the antiglycemic properties of vinegar in healthy adults." *Annals of Nutrition and Metabolism* 56 (1): 74–9.
11. Lukasik, J., M. L. Bradley, T. M. Scott, M. Dea, A. Koo, W. Y. Hsu, J. A. Bartz, and S. R. Farrah. 2003. "Reduction of poliovirus 1, bacteriophages, Salmonella montevideo, and Escherichia coli O157:H7 on strawberries by physical and disinfectant washes." *Journal of Food Protection* 66 (2): 188–93.
12. Rogawansamy, Senthaamarai, Sharyn Gaskin, Michael Taylor, and Dino Pisaniello. 2015. "An evaluation of antifungal agents for the treatment of fungal contamination in indoor air environments." *International Journal of Environmental Research and Public Health* 12 (6): 6319–32.
13. The New York Food Museum. Available at http://www.nyfoodmuseum.org.

14. Budak, N. H., D. Kumbul Doguc, C. M. Savas, A. C. Seydim, T. Kok Tas, M. I. Ciris, and Z. B. Guzel-Seydim. 2011. "Effects of apple cider vinegars produced with different techniques on blood lipids in high-cholesterol-fed rats." *Journal of Agricultural and Food Chemistry* 59: 6638–44.

15. Kim, S. H., C. D. Jun, K. Suk, B. J. Choi, H. Lim, S. Park, S. H. Lee, H. Y. Shin, D. K. Kim, and T. Y. Shin. 2006. "Gallic acid inhibits histamine release and pro-inflammatory cytokine production in mast cells." *Toxicological Sciences* 91 (1): 123–31.

16. Budak, "Effects of apple cider vinegars produced with different techniques on blood lipids in high-cholesterol-fed rats."

17. Kim, "Gallic acid inhibits histamine release and pro-inflammatory cytokine production in mast cells."

18. Shishehbor, "Apple cider vinegar attenuates lipid profile in normal and diabetic rats."

19. Laranjinha, J. A., L. M. Almeida, and V. M. Madeira. 1994. "Reactivity of dietary phenolic acids with peroxyl radicals: antioxidant activity upon low density lipoprotein peroxidation." *Biochemical Pharmacology* 48: 487–94.

20. Kim, "Gallic acid inhibits histamine release and pro-inflammatory cytokine production in mast cells."

21. Johnston, "Vinegar: medicinal uses and antiglycemic effect."

22. Nishino, H., M. Murakoshi, X. Y. Mou, S. Wada, M. Masuda, Y. Ohsaka, Y. Satomi, and K. Jinno. 2005. "Cancer prevention by phytochemicals." *Oncology* 69 (Suppl 1): 38–40.

23. Fu, Hong, Ying Qiang Shi, and Shan Jin Mo. 2004. "Effect of short-chain fatty acids on the proliferation and differentiation of the human colonic adenocarcinoma cell line Caco-2." *Chinese Journal of Digestive Diseases* 5 (3): 115–7.

24. Seki, T., S. Morimura, T. Shigematsu, H. Maeda, and K. Kida. 2004. "Antitumor activity of rice-shochu post-distillation slurry and vinegar produced from the post-distillation slurry via oral administration in a mouse model." *Biofactors* 22 (1–4): 103–5.

25. Mota, A. C., R. D. de Castro, J. de Araújo Oliveira, and E. de Oliveira Lima. 2015. "Antifungal activity of apple cider vinegar on Candida species involved in denture stomatitis." *Journal of Prosthodontics* 24 (4): 296–302.

26. Pinto, T. M., A. C. Neves, M. V. Leão, and A. O. Jorge. 2008. "Vinegar as an antimicrobial agent for control of Candida spp. in complete denture wearers." *Journal of Applied Oral Science* 16 (6): 385–90.

27. Johnston, "Examination of the antiglycemic properties of vinegar in healthy adults."

28. Johnston, C. S., C. M. Kim, and A. J. Buller. 2004. "Vinegar improves insulin sensitivity to a high-carbohydrate meal in subjects with insulin resistance or type 2 diabetes." *Diabetes Care* 27 (1): 281–2.

29. Liljeberg, H., and I. Björck. 1998. "Delayed gastric emptying rate may explain improved glycaemia in healthy subjects to a starchy meal with added vinegar." *European Journal of Clinical Nutrition* 52 (5): 368–71.

30. Entani, E., M. Asai, S. Tsujihata, Y. Tsukamoto, and M. Ohta. 1998. "Antibacterial action of vinegar against food-borne pathogenic bacteria including Escherichia coli O157:H7." *Journal of Food Protection* 61 (8): 953–9.

31. Aziz, N. H., S. E. Farag, L. A. Mousa, and M. A. Abo-Zaid. 1998. "Comparative antibacterial and antifungal effects of some phenolic compounds." *Microbios* 93 (374): 43–54.

32. Bauers, Sandy. "Stronger Vinegar for Greener Cleaning." Philly.com, June 25, 2012. http://www.philly.com/philly/columnists/sandy_bauers/20120625_Stronger_vinegar_for_greener_cleaning.html.

33. Xibib, S., H. Meilan, H. Moller, H. S. Evans, D. Dixin, D. Wenjie, and L. Jianbang. 2003. "Risk factors for oesophageal cancer in Linzhou, China: a case-control study." *Asian Pacific Journal of Cancer Prevention* 4 (2): 119–24.

34. Johnston, "Examination of the antiglycemic properties of vinegar in healthy adults."

35. Johnston, "Vinegar improves insulin sensitivity to a high-carbohydrate meal in subjects with insulin resistance or type 2 diabetes."

36. Setorki, M., S. Asgary, A. Eidi, A. H. Rohani, and M. Khazaei. 2010. "Acute effects of vinegar intake on some biochemical risk factors of atherosclerosis in hypercholesterolemic rabbits." *Lipids in Health and Disease* 9: 10.

37. Ostman, E., Y. Granfeldt, L. Persson, I. Björck. 2005. "Vinegar supplementation lowers glucose and insulin responses and increases satiety after a bread meal in healthy subjects." *European Journal of Clinical Nutrition* 59 (9): 983–8.

38. Johnston, C. S., and A. J. Buller. 2005. "Vinegar and peanut products as complementary foods to reduce postprandial glycemia." *Journal of the American Dietetic Association* 105 (12): 1939–42.

39. Russell, I. J., J. E. Michalek, J. D. Flechas, and G. E. Abraham. 1995. "Treatment of fibromyalgia syndrome with Super Malic: a randomized, double blind, placebo controlled, crossover pilot study." *Journal of Rheumatology* 22 (5): 953–8.

40. Abraham, Guy E., and Jorge D. Flechas. 1992. "Management of fibromyalgia: rationale for the use of magnesium and malic acid." *Journal of Nutritional Medicine* 3 (1): 49–59.

41. Locatelli, Claudriana, Fabíola Branco Filippin-Monteiro, Ariana Centa, and Tânia Beatriz Creczinsky-Pasa. 2013. "Antioxidant, antitumoral and anti-inflammatory activities of gallic acid." In *Handbook on Gallic Acid: Natural Occurrences, Antioxidant Properties and Health Implications*, edited by Michelle A. Thompson and Parker B. Collins, 215–30. Hauppage, NY: Nova Science Publishers.

42. Baroody, Theodore A. 1991. *Alkalize or Die: Superior Health through Proper Alkaline-Acid Balance*. Waynesville, NC: Holographic Health, Inc.

43. Jung, H. H., S. D. Sho, C. K. Yoo, H. H. Lim, and S. W. Chae. 2002. "Vinegar treatment in the management of granular myringitis." *The Journal of Laryngology & Otology* 116 (3): 176–80.

44. Shishehbor, "Apple cider vinegar attenuates lipid profile in normal and diabetic rats."

45. Budak, "Effects of apple cider vinegars produced with different techniques on blood lipids in high-cholesterol-fed rats."

46. White, Andrea M., and Carol S. Johnston. 2007. "Vinegar ingestion at bedtime moderates waking glucose concentrations in adults with well-controlled type 2 diabetes." *Diabetes Care* 30 (11): 2814–5.

47. Johnston, "Examination of the antiglycemic properties of vinegar in healthy adults."

48. Van Dijk, A. E., M. R. Olthof, J. C. Meeuse, E. Seebus, R. J. Heine, and R. M. van Dam. 2009. "Acute effects of decaffeinated coffee and the major coffee components chlorogenic acid and trigonelline on glucose tolerance." *Diabetes Care* 32 (6): 1023–5.

49. Liljeberg, "Delayed gastric emptying rate may explain improved glycaemia in healthy subjects to a starchy meal with added vinegar."

50. Tanaka, Hiroko, Kenichi Watanabe, Meilei Ma, Masao Hirayama, Takashi Kobayashi, Hiroshi Oyama, Yoshiko Sakaguchi, Mitsuo Kanda, Makoto Kodama, and Yoshifusa Aizawa. 2009. "The effects of γ -aminobutyric acid, vinegar, and dried bonito on blood pressure in normotensive and mildly or moderately hypertensive volunteers." *Journal of Clinical Biochemistry and Nutrition* 45 (1): 93–100.

51. Kondo, S., K. Tayama, Y. Tsukamoto, K. Ikeda, and Y. Yamori. 2001. "Antihypertensive effects of acetic acid and vinegar on spontaneously hypertensive rats." *Bioscience, Biotechnology, and Biochemistry* 65 (12): 2690–4.

52. Watanabe, T., Y. Arai, Y. Mitsui, T. Kusaura, W. Okawa, Y. Kajihara, and I. Saito. 2006. "The blood pressure-lowering effect and safety of chlorogenic acid from green coffee bean extract in essential hypertension." *Clinical and Experimental Hypertension* 28 (5): 439–49.

53. Entani, "Antibacterial action of vinegar against food-borne pathogenic bacteria including Escherichia coli O157:H7."

54. Aziz, "Comparative antibacterial and antifungal effects of some phenolic compounds."

55. Mindell, Earl. 2002. *Amazing Apple Cider Vinegar*. New York, NY: McGraw-Hill Education.

56. Trinidad, T. P., T. M. Wolever, and L. U. Thompson. 1996. "Effect of acetate and propionate on calcium absorption from the rectum and distal colon of humans." *The American Journal of Clinical Nutrition* 63 (4): 574–8.

57. Kishi, M., M. Fukaya, Y. Tsukamoto, T. Nagasawa, K. Takehana, and N. Nishizawa. 1999. "Enhancing effect of dietary vinegar on the intestinal absorption of calcium in ovariectomized rats." *Bioscience, Biotechnology, and Biochemistry* 63 (5): 905–10.

58. Yoon, Chong-Hyeon, Soo-Jin Chung, Sang-Won Lee, Yong-Beom Park, Soo-Kon Lee, and Min-Chan Park. 2013. "Gallic acid, a natural polyphenolic acid, induces apoptosis and inhibits proinflammatory gene expressions in rheumatoid arthritis fibroblast-like synoviocytes." *Joint Bone Spine* 80 (3): 274–9.

59. Yucel Sengun, I., and M. Karapinar. 2005. "Effectiveness of household natural sanitizers in the elimination of Salmonella typhimurium on rocket (Eruca sativa Miller) and spring onion (Allium cepa L.)." *International Journal of Food Microbiology* 98 (3): 319–23.

60. Kim, "Gallic acid inhibits histamine release and pro-inflammatory cytokine production in mast cells."

61. Ibid.

62. Kaushik, V., T. Malik, and S. R. Saeed. 2010. "Interventions for acute otitis externa." *The Cochrane Database of Systematic Reviews* (1): CD004740.

63. Mindell, *Amazing Apple Cider Vinegar*.

64. Atik, Derya, Cem Atik, and Celalettin Karatepe. 2016. "The effect of external apple vinegar application on varicosity symptoms, pain, and social appearance anxiety: a randomized controlled trial." *Evidence-Based Complementary and Alternative Medicine* 2016: 6473678.

65. Kilfoil Jr., Roger Lee, Garry Shtofmakher, Gregory Taylor, and Jessica Botvinick. 2014. "Acetic acid iontophoresis for the treatment of insertional Achilles tendonitis." *BMJ Case Reports* July (1): 1–3.

66. Johnston, "Examination of the antiglycemic properties of vinegar in healthy adults."

67. Johnston, "Vinegar improves insulin sensitivity to a high-carbohydrate meal in subjects with insulin resistance or type 2 diabetes."

68. Liljeberg, "Delayed gastric emptying rate may explain improved glycaemia in healthy subjects to a starchy meal with added vinegar."

69. Japour, C. J., R. Vohra, P. K. Vohra, L. Garfunkel, and N. Chin. 1999. "Management of heel pain syndrome with acetic acid iontophoresis." *Journal of the American Podiatric Medical Association* 89 (5): 251–7.

70. Osborne, H. R., and G. T. Allison. 2006. "Treatment of plantar fasciitis by LowDye taping and iontophoresis: short term results of a double blinded, randomised, placebo controlled clinical trial of dexamethasone and acetic acid." *British Journal of Sports Medicine* 40 (6): 545–9.

71. Russell, "Treatment of fibromyalgia syndrome with Super Malic."

72. Abraham, "Management of fibromyalgia."

73. Salovaara, Susan, Ann-Sofie Sandberg, and Thomas Andlid. 2002. "Organic acids influence iron uptake in the human epithelial cell line Caco-2." *Journal of Agricultural and Food Chemistry* 50 (21): 6233–8.

74. Kim, "Gallic acid inhibits histamine release and pro-inflammatory cytokine production in mast cells."

75. Ibid.

76. Cropley, V., R. Croft, B. Silber, C. Neale, A. Scholey, C. Stough, and J. Schmitt. 2012. "Does coffee enriched with chlorogenic acids improve mood and cognition after acute administration in healthy elderly? A pilot study." *Psychopharmacology (Berl)* 219 (3): 737–49.

77. Liljeberg, "Delayed gastric emptying rate may explain improved glycaemia in healthy subjects to a starchy meal with added vinegar."

78. Johnston, "Examination of the antiglycemic properties of vinegar in healthy adults."

79. Johnston, "Vinegar improves insulin sensitivity to a high-carbohydrate meal in subjects with insulin resistance or type 2 diabetes."

80. Liljeberg, "Delayed gastric emptying rate may explain improved glycaemia in healthy subjects to a starchy meal with added vinegar."

81. Salovaara, "Organic acids influence iron uptake in the human epithelial cell line Caco-2."

82. Abraham, "Management of fibromyalgia: rationale for the use of magnesium and malic Acid."

83. Sadeghi, Masoumeh, Mazdak Khalili, Masoud Pourmoghaddas, and Mohammad Talaei. 2012. "The correlation between blood pressure and hot flashes in menopausal women." *ARYA Atherosclerosis* 8 (1): 32–5.

84. Kondo, "Antihypertensive effects of acetic acid and vinegar on spontaneously hypertensive rats."

85. Watanabe, "The blood pressure-lowering effect and safety of chlorogenic acid from green coffee bean extract in essential hypertension."

86. Shaw, Terri. 2003. "Peru tries vinegar against cervical cancer." *Bulletin of the World Health Organization* 81 (1): 73–4.

87. University of Zimbabwe/JHPIEGO Cervical Cancer Project. 1999. "Visual inspection with acetic acid for cervical-cancer screening: test qualities in a primary-care setting." *Lancet* 353 (9156): 869–73.

88. Kashimura, J., M. Kimura, and Y. Itokawa. 1996. "The effects of isomaltulose, isomalt, and isomaltulose-based oligomers on mineral absorption and retention." *Biological Trace Element Research* 54 (3): 239–50.

89. Salovaara, "Organic acids influence iron uptake in the human epithelial cell line Caco-2."

90. Perkins, R. Allen, and Shannon S. Morgan. 2004. "Poisoning, envenomation, and trauma from marine creatures." *American Family Physician* 69 (4): 885–90.

91. Johnston, "Vinegar improves insulin sensitivity to a high-carbohydrate meal in subjects with insulin resistance or type 2 diabetes."

92. Fukami, H., H. Tachimoto, M. Kishi, T. Kaga, Y. Tanaka, Y. Koga, and T. Shirasawa. 2009. "Continuous ingestion of acetic acid bacteria: effect on cognitive function in healthy middle-aged and elderly persons." *Anti-Aging Medicine* 6 (7): 60–5.

93. Trinidad, "Effect of acetate and propionate on calcium absorption from the rectum and distal colon of humans."

94. Kishi, "Enhancing effect of dietary vinegar on the intestinal absorption of calcium in ovariectomized rats."

95. Kashimura, "The effects of isomaltulose, isomalt, and isomaltulose-based oligomers on mineral absorption and retention."

96. Salovaara, "Organic acids influence iron uptake in the human epithelial cell line Caco-2."

97. Kashimura, "The effects of isomaltulose, isomalt, and isomaltulose-based oligomers on mineral absorption and retention."

98. Salovaara, "Organic acids influence iron uptake in the human epithelial cell line Caco-2."

99. Osborne, "Treatment of plantar fasciitis by LowDye taping and iontophoresis."

100. The Online Archive of American Folk Medicine, http://ahrt.ucla.edu.

101. Lukasik, "Reduction of poliovirus 1, bacteriophages, Salmonella montevideo, and Escherichia coli O157:H7 on strawberries by physical and disinfectant washes."

102. Aziz, "Comparative antibacterial and antifungal effects of some phenolic compounds."

103. Johnston, "Examination of the antiglycemic properties of vinegar in healthy adults."

104. Bilardi, Jade, Sandra Walker, Ruth McNair, Julie Mooney-Somers, Meredith Temple-Smith, Clare Bellhouse, Christopher Fairley, Marcus Chen, and Catriona Bradshaw. 2016. "Women's management of recurrent bacterial vaginosis and experiences of clinical care: a qualitative study." *PLOS One* 11 (3): e0151794.

105. Mota, "Antifungal activity of apple cider vinegar on Candida species involved in denture stomatitis."

106. Salovaara, "Organic acids influence iron uptake in the human epithelial cell line Caco-2."

107. Johnston, "Vinegar and peanut products as complementary foods to reduce postprandial glycemia."

108. Kondo, T., M. Kishi, T. Fushimi, S. Ugajin, and T. Kaga. 2009. "Vinegar intake reduces body weight, body fat mass, and serum triglyceride levels in obese Japanese subjects." *Bioscience, Biotechnology, and Biochemistry* 73 (8): 1837–43.

109. Mota, "Antifungal activity of apple cider vinegar on Candida species involved in denture stomatitis."

110. Lukasik, "Reduction of poliovirus 1, bacteriophages, Salmonella montevideo, and Escherichia coli O157:H7 on strawberries by physical and disinfectant washes."

111. Yucel Sengun, "Effectiveness of household natural sanitizers in the elimination of Salmonella typhimurium on rocket (Eruca sativa Miller) and spring onion (Allium cepa L.)."

112. Basson, N. J., A. N. Quick, and C. J. Thomas. 1992. "Household products as sanitising agents in denture cleansing." *The Journal of the Dental Association of South Africa* 47 (10): 437–9.

113. Pinto, "Vinegar as an antimicrobial agent for control of Candida spp. in complete denture wearers."

114. Kennedy, Liz. "Is Tooth Whitening Safe?" *Reader's Digest.* http://www.rd.com/health/beauty/is-tooth-whitening-safe/?_ga=1.130248335.1845637712.1486984392.

115 . Ullah, Aziz. "The Remediation of Urine." Cleanfax.com. http://www.cleanfax.com/diversification/the-remediation-of-urine/.

116. Steinemann, Anne C., Ian C. MacGregor, Sydney M. Gordon, Lisa G. Gallagher, Amy L. Davis, Daniel S. Ribeiro, and Lance A. Wallace. 2016. "Fragranced consumer products: Chemicals emitted, ingredients unlisted." *Air Quality, Atmosphere & Health* 9 (8): 861–6.

117. Smith-Spangler, C., M. L. Brandeau, G. E. Hunter, J. C. Bavinger, M. Pearson, P. J. Eschbach, V. Sundaram, H. Liu, P. Schirmer, C. Stave, I. Olkin, and D. M. Bravata. 2012. "Are organic foods safer or healthier than conventional alternatives? A systematic review." *Annals of Internal Medicine* 157 (5): 348–66.

ABOUT THE AUTHOR

SUSAN BRANSON earned an undergraduate degree in biology from St. Francis Xavier University, then a MSc in toxicology from the University of Ottawa. From there, she worked in research: in the field, in the lab, as a writer, and as an administrator. She took time off and stayed at home after her second child was born. In addition to being a stay-at-home mom, she also took violin lessons, photography courses, earned a diploma in writing, and ultimately became a holistic nutritionist. Susan is a member of CSNN's Alumni Association, Canada's leading holistic nutrition school.

ABOUT FAMILIUS

VISIT OUR WEBSITE: WWW.FAMILIUS.COM

JOIN OUR FAMILY

There are lots of ways to connect with us! Subscribe to our news-letters at www.familius.com to receive uplifting daily inspiration, essays from our Pater Familius, a free ebook every month, and the first word on special discounts and Familius news.

GET BULK DISCOUNTS

If you feel a few friends and family might benefit from what you've read, let us know and we'll be happy to provide you with quantity discounts. Simply email us at orders@familius.com.

CONNECT

Facebook: www.facebook.com/paterfamilius
Twitter: @familiustalk, @paterfamilius1
Pinterest: www.pinterest.com/familius
Instagram: @familiustalk

FAMILIUS

> THE MOST IMPORTANT WORK YOU
> EVER DO WILL BE WITHIN THE
> WALLS OF YOUR OWN HOME.